Canvas of Courage

The Art of Healing, Hope, and Gratitude for Young Mothers Facing Cancer

Nerissa Balland

Canvas of Courage Press

Canvas of Courage

Copyright © 2026 by Nerissa Balland

ISBN 979-8-218-92451-5 (paperback)

All rights reserved. No part of this publication may be reproduced, scanned or transmitted in any form, digital or printed, without the written permission of the author.

First Edition: 2026

Published by Canvas of Courage Press

Fort Lauderdale, FL 33328

United States

www.nerissaballand.com

NO AI TRAINING: Any use of this publication to "train" generative artificial intelligence (AI) technologies is prohibited.

Cover Illustration: Nerissa Balland

To my husband, **Michael**—
my steady ground, my fiercest advocate, my quiet strength.
Thank you for standing beside me when fear was loud,
for believing in me when I struggled to believe in myself,
and for loving me with patience, humor, and unwavering devotion.
I could not have walked this path without you.

To my children, **Eli and Teddy**—
the greatest gifts of my life.
Being your mother is my most sacred role,
one I hold with humility, reverence, and fierce love.
Through you, I learned what unconditional love truly means.
You make life worth fighting for—every single day.

And to my Cancer Coach, **Leslie Kelly**—
thank you for your guidance, your honesty, and your unwavering presence.
For pushing me on the days I believed I could not take another step.
For giving me the tools, the language, and the wisdom
to stand back up when I could barely breathe.
Your work changed my life more than you will ever know.

Contents

The First Layer *Introduction*	1
Brushstrokes of Grace *Sadie's Story*	4
The Music Between the Moments *Stephanie's Story*	11
The Art of Embracing Cancer *Nerissa's Story*	17
The Art of Returning to Yourself *Alicia's Story*	27
The Art of Returning to Life *Christina's Story*	34
The Art of Learning to Feel the Sun Again *Colleen's Story*	47
The Art of Holding On, One Step at a Time *Liz's Story*	55
The Art of Showing Up *Jennifer's Story*	66
The Art of Rising Again *Julia's Story*	78
The Art of Rising in the Ruins *Keilymar's Story*	83
The Art of Carrying a Baby and a Diagnosis at the Same Time *Michelle's Story*	94
The Art of Being Held *Shauna's Story*	107
The Art of Trusting Your Inner Voice *Chelsea's Story*	115
The Art of Ordinary Miracles *Nicole's Story*	133
The Art of Holding Two Lives *Maria's Story*	145

The Art of Permission *Sara's Story*	152
The Art of Living Out Loud *Stephanie's Story*	158
The Art of Holding On and Letting Go *Carrie's Story*	165
The Art of Becoming Unbreakable *Melanie's Story*	180
The Healing Science of Art	186
An Invitation to Create	192
What We Carry Forward	195
About the Author	199
Acknowledgments	201

The First Layer
Introduction

I f you found your way here, I want you to know something before you read a single story: You are not late. You are not lost. And you are not alone.

Books like this are rarely picked up by accident. They are found in waiting rooms and quiet bedrooms, during sleepless nights and long afternoons. They are opened by women searching for language when words feel just out of reach — by mothers, daughters, caregivers, survivors, and those still in the middle of it all.

This book does not promise answers. It does not offer formulas or timelines or guarantees. What it offers instead is presence.

Like the first layer of paint on a canvas, this beginning is not meant to be perfect or complete. It is meant to hold. To prepare space. To soften the surface so that what comes next can be received.

Nerissa Balland

. . .

Canvas of Courage was born from listening — deeply and without interruption — to women whose lives were irrevocably changed by diagnosis. Women who did not ask to become experts in fear, resilience, grief, or grace, yet found themselves fluent in all four. Women who mothered through uncertainty. Who learned how to live while carrying the unthinkable. Who discovered that healing is not a finish line, but a practice.

This book is not about fighting cancer.
    It is about *living with it*.
    Living through it.
    Living after it.
    And for some, learning how to live alongside its shadow.

Each chapter you are about to read is a life — layered, textured, unfinished in the most human way. Some stories end in remission. Some continue in uncertainty. Some are written in the present tense, others in memory. All of them are true. All of them matter.

You will notice something as you move through these pages:
    No two journeys are the same.
    And yet — there are echoes.

You will hear familiar fears. Familiar questions. Familiar guilt, anger, tenderness, and love. You may see yourself reflected in moments you didn't know how to name until now. You may feel comforted, unsettled, inspired, or undone. All of that is welcome here.

This book is not meant to be rushed.
You do not need to read it cover to cover.
You do not need to be "ready."
Some chapters may feel like a mirror.
Others may feel like a hand reaching back for yours.
Pause when you need to.
Skip ahead.
Return later.
Reread a story if it's the one that speaks to you.
Healing does not happen all at once.
Neither does understanding.
Neither does hope.
Like art, healing happens in layers —
some visible, some buried, some revealed slowly.

This first layer is simply an opening.
    A breath.
    A moment of acknowledgment.
    You are here.
    And that, in itself, is enough to begin.

Brushstrokes of Grace
Sadie's Story

H*ealing doesn't always look like a fight. Sometimes, it looks like surrender.*

"Grace isn't passive—it's power in soft form. It's the art of standing still while everything inside you trembles, of painting peace where fear once lived."

The mind learns in thunderclaps—and keeps its wisdom in whispers.

For Sadie, the thunder came in the word itself: *cancer*.

The whisper followed in the form of a stranger's voice—soft, unexpected, unforgettable:

"Don't make enemies with what's inside you."

That one sentence changed everything.

Sadie was twenty-nine when her world shifted. A young mother of two girls, six and three, she had no family history of breast cancer. She was busy with work, motherhood, and all the invisible labor of caring for others. She had already known what vigilance felt like—

years earlier, she had discovered a lump while breastfeeding, one that turned out to be a clogged duct. So, when she felt something new, years later, beneath her arm in the shower, she wanted desperately to believe it was nothing. The holidays were coming. Her husband's birthday was near. Life was too full to stop.

But the lump grew. Her gut whispered what her mind refused to admit: *This is different.*

The Cyclone Begins

Everything after that moved in fast-forward. Appointments blurred together—scans, biopsies, doctors whose faces she can still recall but whose words sometimes dissolve into static. It was Valentine's Day when she lay on the imaging table, gel on her chest, the machine humming above. She had searched the internet for what cancer might look like on a sonogram—those jagged, uneven edges that don't belong—and she recognized them in the grayscale shadows before the technician even spoke.

The doctor left the room, came back, and asked if they could biopsy immediately. Sadie wasn't ready. "It's Valentine's Day," she remembers thinking. "I just want to go home."

Days later, the call came.

The voice on the other end confirmed what she already knew in her bones—but knowing and hearing are two different earthquakes.

She was diagnosed with triple-positive breast cancer, stage IIA.

Her first thought wasn't *me*. It was *my girls*.

The Nail Salon Stranger

. . .

For days, Sadie floated in a fog of denial. She told no one at first, not even her mother or sisters, whom she loved dearly. "Saying it out loud made it real," she said later. "And I wasn't ready for it to be real."

She remembers going to a nail salon—a small, ordinary act of distraction. There, she met a woman who radiated confidence and warmth, the kind of person who seems to carry sunlight in her posture. They talked about travel, about life. As Sadie was leaving, the woman smiled and said, "Book the trip. Go."

"I can't," Sadie replied quietly. "I have breast cancer."

The woman took her hand, looked directly into her eyes, and said, "You're going to be okay. Don't make enemies with what's inside you. Befriend it."

It felt absurd at first, even offensive. But those words followed her home and began to root in her. They became the beginning of a transformation. Sadie realized that denial was a form of war—an endless fight with herself. Acceptance, she discovered, was not weakness; it was peace.

Parenting Through Treatment

When treatment began—six cycles of chemotherapy, Herceptin, and a five-year pill regimen—Sadie's life revolved around her children. Every schedule was built around pickups, school lunches, and bedtime hugs. Her goal was simple but sacred: to make life feel as normal as possible for her daughters.

On her first treatment day, she refused to let anyone else pick up her children. "I wanted them to see me there, smiling, so they wouldn't think cancer took me away."

As the treatments progressed, fatigue deepened, and asking for help became a new kind of courage. Her mother-in-law moved downstairs and cooked dinner each night. Her husband cleaned, often for the first time. Sadie, who had always taken pride in doing everything herself, learned to release control. "I used to think asking for help made me weak," she said. "But it turns out pretending I didn't need help was the real weakness."

Her oldest daughter, then seven, began saying, "Mommy, my heart hurts." Sadie didn't recognize it at first—it wasn't physical. It was anxiety. The invisible echo of fear that rippled through the house even when no one said the word *cancer*.

Sadie did what she could. She explained gently that the medicine was strong, that it would help her, but it might make her look sick. She let her daughters cut her hair shorter and shorter until it was gone. They wrinkled their noses, laughed, cried, called her "silly." She smiled with them, even as she swallowed her tears.

"When I lost my eyebrows and lashes," she said, "that's when I finally looked like I had cancer. That was the hardest part."

The Panic and the Promise

After her first chemo session, Sadie had a panic attack. Her heart raced; her breath shortened. She thought she might die. When she told her doctor, he offered Xanax. She refused. "I didn't want another pill. I wanted hope."

A few days later, a friend called and offered her something else— a small bottle of CBD oil left behind by her late father-in-law. Sadie took ten drops. Ten minutes later, she was standing, eating pineapple, laughing with her kids. "It was my sign," she said. "That's when I knew I could do this."

It didn't erase her pain or exhaustion, but it reminded her that relief was possible. That joy could still find her.

. . .

The Art of Healing

As her body healed, Sadie began to heal her mind. She started watching documentaries—stories about people who had overcome illness through mindset, meditation, and emotional awareness. She discovered spiritual teachers like Sadhguru and the documentary *Heal*. She began to believe that the mind could make the body sick—and that the mind could also help it recover.

"Cancer was the mirror," she said. "It showed me the life I was living wasn't the one I wanted. I was always people-pleasing, worrying, saying yes when I meant no. My body finally said stop."

That realization brought freedom, not guilt. She started meditating. Walking barefoot outside. Listening—really listening—to the quiet voice within her. Gratitude became her medicine.

"Before cancer, I didn't really *see* my life," she said. "Now I wake up and feel it. Even just opening my eyes feels like a blessing."

Sadie began to see herself as an artist—not just in the literal sense, but in the act of shaping her inner landscape. She painted each day with gentleness: music, prayer, warm baths, sunlight. Acceptance was her brush. Gratitude was her color. Together, they became her art of living.

Motherhood Reimagined

Parenting after cancer carried a new gravity. Sadie still worries about her daughter's lingering sadness, still notices when her eyes look far away. She's learned to meet those moments not with guilt but with curiosity. "If your sadness had a color, what would it be?" she asks gently.

She's teaching her children—through her own example—that

strength doesn't always roar. Sometimes it hums quietly between breaths, between tears, between chemo rounds and laughter.

"I used to think I had to be brave for them," she said. "Now I realize, being real with them was the bravest thing."

A Graceful Transformation

When asked what cancer gave her—what gift it left behind—Sadie pauses. "It made me feel alive," she finally says. "Really alive. Before, I didn't know how lucky I was just to wake up."

Her days are slower now, more intentional. Gratitude lives in the smallest corners of her home—the warmth of sunlight through a window, the laughter of her girls, the smell of dinner cooking downstairs.

Sadie no longer calls it a battle. She calls it a becoming.

Cancer was the brush. Grace was the paint.

And life—this unfinished, ever-changing canvas—is still her masterpiece.

Closing Reflection

What we resist, we feed with fear. What we embrace, we begin to heal.

Sadie's story reminds us that grace is not the absence of struggle—it's the posture we hold inside it. Through motherhood, she learned that love isn't always loud. Through illness, she learned that surrender is not defeat. It's trust.

. . .

Sadie's Grace Notes

- **Trust your intuition.** If something feels wrong, it probably is. Listen. Act.
- **Ask for help early.** It's not weakness—it's wisdom. Healing is communal.
- **Talk to your children honestly.** They feel everything. Offer gentle truth.
- **Name emotions with color.** "If your sadness had a color, what would it be?" opens more than "What's wrong?" ever could.
- **Micro-gratitude.** Three small thanks before bed: a laugh, a taste, a scent.
- **Comfort rituals.** Epsom baths, soft music, CBD, breathing, and light. Small acts, sacred power.
- **Release guilt.** You are healing. That's your work right now.
- **Reframe the language.** You are not fighting cancer—you're learning from it.
- **Remember your body is listening.** Speak to it kindly.
- **Teach your children grace through example.** Let them see you rest. Let them see you rise.

The Music Between the Moments
Stephanie's Story

Sometimes the quietest songs carry the loudest strength.

Art, at its core, is rhythm — the pulse beneath the surface that keeps us moving, even when the world feels heavy with silence. Some rhythms are painted, some are written, and others are sung softly in the space between struggle and surrender. When I first spoke with Stephanie, I heard her rhythm long before I saw it — a melody of courage wrapped in gratitude, keeping time against fear.

Her story, like a song painted on canvas, carries both light and shadow: the deep notes of loss, the high tones of laughter, and a steady beat of motherhood that plays no matter what storms arrive. In Stephanie's music, healing isn't loud. It's steady — a hum of grace that rises each morning with her daughters, two small mirrors of love who remind her what every note is for.

. . .

Nerissa Balland

The Music Between the Moments

When Stephanie was first told she had *primary thyroid lymphoma* at 37, her world went quiet. It was an incidental discovery — her doctor, during a routine exam, noticed something different in her thyroid nodules. The biopsy that followed delivered the kind of news that rearranges everything.

She underwent fifteen rounds of radiation, watching her world shrink to treatment rooms and scan reports. But she kept moving, kept mothering, kept showing up for life. The rhythm of survival began as a whisper — a quiet insistence that this would not be her final song.

Then, just a year later, the melody changed again.

At 38, she found a lump during a self-exam — the kind of moment that stops all sound. Having already watched her sister battle breast cancer, she hoped this was nothing. But the biopsy revealed *invasive ductal carcinoma*, stage IIIA. All her lymph nodes were positive. Suddenly, she wasn't just a mother of two — she was a mother fighting two different cancers in two different years.

And yet, when she talks about that time, her voice is calm, almost lyrical.

"I've been lucky," she says. "I have the most amazing support system of anybody out there — my ER nurse friends, my family, my coworkers. I don't know how people do this without them."

Her gratitude doesn't come from denial; it comes from clarity. She knows how fragile everything is. Working as a nurse in an emergency room, she has seen how quickly life can change. "We see how fragile it all is," she told me. "So I just take the day I'm given. I try to make it a good one."

During her eight rounds of chemotherapy — four rounds of AC and four rounds of Taxol — she let the noise of the hospital fade into the background and found her own kind of music: *Kenny Chesney, Netflix, laughter.* Sometimes it was her mom sitting beside her; sometimes it was friends stopping by the chemo room like it was a backstage pass to strength. She turned treatment into connection — a rhythm of resilience in a place built for endurance.

Motherhood in the Key of Grace

Stephanie has two daughters: an eight-year-old and a two-year-old. When she speaks of them, her voice softens into something sacred.

She didn't hide her diagnosis from her older daughter. Together, they read books about cancer from the American Cancer Society and Amazon, learning how to talk about what was happening. "We were open, but gentle," she says. "She needed to know that Mommy was doing everything she could to be healthy again."

The younger one, just a toddler, became a mirror for surrender. "I knew she wouldn't remember this time," Stephanie explains. "So I let myself ask for help." Her honesty about this feels revolutionary — a reminder that strength isn't always self-sufficiency. Sometimes it's the grace to say *yes* when someone offers to fold your laundry, drive your child to daycare, or sit with you while you rest.

She laughs about "mom guilt," that invisible weight carried by so many mothers facing treatment. "You have to let it go," she says. "Your child doesn't need you perfect — they need you present."

The Sound of Healing

When support groups didn't quite fit — mostly older women whose life stage was worlds apart from hers — Stephanie found solace elsewhere: in sound and stillness.

She discovered a local float spa, where the weightlessness of Epsom-salt water became its own kind of therapy — a suspended moment of peace. She paired that with music: *Kenny Chesney, country anthems, soft melodies that mirrored her heartbeat.*

Music became medicine. "I don't think I would've survived without it," she said, laughing. It wasn't just background noise — it was a language of permission. Permission to cry. Permission to smile. Permission to live.

Her playlist became a palette — songs as brushstrokes, filling the empty spaces between fear and faith. On days she felt strong, she sang along. On days she couldn't, she simply let the music hold her.

A Life Rewritten in Color and Sound

Cancer didn't make Stephanie grateful overnight. It broke her open, rearranged her priorities, and gave her back to herself piece by piece. "I didn't look at cancer as a gift," she says. "But I look at all the things I've gained from it as the gift."

Now she no longer waits to live. She books the trip. She goes to concerts with her daughter. She plans girls' weekends and eats dessert first. "I can make more money later," she says, "but I can't make more memories if I don't go now."

Her words echo like a chorus of defiance and devotion. She's living life in vivid color — not because the pain disappeared, but because she decided not to mute the joy.

Closing Reflection

. . .

When I listen to Stephanie's story, I hear harmony — the kind that happens when gratitude meets grace. Her strength isn't measured in volume or perfection, but in her willingness to keep singing even when the melody shifts.

In my own healing journey, I've come to believe that art and music are twin languages of survival. They ask nothing but presence. Stephanie's art is her rhythm — the way she chooses to dance through difficulty, to turn exhaustion into tenderness, and fear into a song that her daughters will one day recognize as love.

Sometimes healing isn't about silence or stillness. It's about finding the music between the moments — and letting gratitude be the echo that lingers.

Stephanie's Grace Notes

- **Accept help — it's not weakness.** Your kids need your energy, not your perfection. Let friends, family, or neighbors assist.
- **Stay honest with your children.** Use age-appropriate books and involve schools or counselors early.
- **Build your circle.** If no local groups exist, use Facebook communities for your specific diagnosis.
- **Make memories, not excuses.** Take the trip, go to the concert, eat the cake. Life is meant to be lived now.
- **Lean on music and self-care.** Floating, massages, playlists — find what soothes your nervous system.
- **Think one inning at a time.** Healing, like baseball, isn't won in the first inning. Take each stage as it comes.
- **Release financial guilt.** You can earn later — but you can't redo the moments that matter most today.

- **Let gratitude lead.** Even small joys — a warm bath, a child's laugh, a song on the radio — are healing art forms.

The Art of Embracing Cancer
Nerissa's Story

Sometimes your greatest challenge awakens an opportunity to become your greatest gift.

There are moments in life that crack you open so completely that the world can never look the same again.

Cancer was that moment for me.

It confronted every truth I avoided, every dream I postponed, every part of myself I had silenced. And yet, within that rupture was an invitation—to return home to myself, to my art, to my purpose, and to the woman I had abandoned long before cancer arrived.

My story is not about fighting.

It is a story about awakening.

Not because it was beautiful.

Not because it was fair.

But because it offered me a second chance at living more authentically.

The Moment the World Split Open

In August of 2016, I was five months pregnant, working from home in Miami Beach, locked indoors during the Zika outbreak. I was on my weekly conference call from my makeshift home office when my phone began to vibrate relentlessly—texts, missed calls, voicemails stacking on top of one another.

My eldest son, Eli, was fifteen months old and enrolled in early childcare. My husband, Michael, was at work. Nothing about that day was supposed to be extraordinary.

Scrolling through the messages, I felt an unease I couldn't yet name. Both my husband and my dermatologist—my good friend, Dr. Lawrence Schiffman—had tried to reach me. Neither left details. Only the same message, over and over:

Call me back as soon as possible.

I called Larry first.

"The biopsy is malignant."

A tiny mole on my back—one I had removed three separate times—had finally revealed its truth.

Melanoma.

The kind of word that steals your breath before you even understand it.

I froze. And then, embarrassed to admit, I felt confused for a split second. Skin cancer didn't feel like *real* cancer. It felt like something you scraped away and moved on from.

I couldn't have been more wrong.

"You need to see an oncologist immediately," Larry said.

In the silence that followed, an entire lifetime echoed inside me.

My grandmother—whom I cared for at nineteen, shaving her legs, helping her dress, watching her smile through pain she refused to let us see.

The artist I once was—the girl who left Pratt Institute with an MFA and a promise to herself that she would create boldly, honestly, fearlessly... until bills, expectations, and fear quieted her voice.

The young woman who traded paintbrushes for promotions, canvases for conference rooms, passion for stability.

And beneath all of that, smaller and softer than everything else, I heard another sound.

A heartbeat.

The impossible heartbeat inside me—the child I fought years of infertility to conceive.

Cancer didn't just shatter my reality.

It tore open every story I carried about motherhood, womanhood, purpose, identity, and worth.

The First Stroke

Within forty-eight hours, I found myself in an oncology waiting room at Sylvester Comprehensive Cancer Center. I waited six hours to be seen. I remember looking around the room, searching for someone who looked like me.

There was no one.

Mostly older patients. Different phases of life. I was thirty-eight, visibly five-and-a-half months pregnant, and terrified.

When I was finally ushered in to see a highly recommended doctor, the appointment lasted less than ten minutes. He would not discuss treatment or next steps unless I was willing to terminate my pregnancy. In his medical opinion, he would not treat me if I remained pregnant.

I walked out in a daze.

I had walked in with hope and left with dread. No one had told me I was dying in that moment. It didn't feel like this was my only option.

My husband and I sought a second opinion.

Within a week, we were sitting with an oncologist and oncology surgeon at Mount Sinai Medical Center in Miami Beach—doctors who looked at me as a whole person, not a liability. That appointment restored something essential: a plan.

I did not need to terminate my pregnancy. But I did need immediate wide excision surgery on my back—without general anesthesia.

I remember lying on my side, propped with pillows, unable to lie face down, awake and painfully still as lidocaine numbed the incision area. When they finished stitching the six-inch vertical incision, I knew this was only the beginning.

The margins were clean.

The next step was waiting.

I carried my baby to thirty-nine weeks. After delivery, I had two to three weeks before nuclear medicine, bilateral sentinel lymph node removal, and the long wait to see whether the cancer had traveled.

When Control Slips Away

The sentinel lymph node biopsy was its own ordeal. While being prepped for surgery, I repeatedly asked the staff to express my lactating breasts while I was under anesthesia so I wouldn't wake in additional pain. A nurse looked confused, then glanced at my chart.

"Aren't you having a double mastectomy?"

My body jolted upright. Panic surged. I began texting my

husband, my mother, my mother-in-law. I refused to be sedated until the surgeon confirmed the paperwork was wrong.

It was.

After surgery, I couldn't return home. Nuclear radiation made it unsafe to be around my newborn and two-year-old. I stayed with my mother in a hotel room—listening to the echo of motherhood just out of reach.

A week later, the call came.

The cancer had traveled—to both underarms.

It was metastatic.

Treatment began: eight months of Keytruda infusions. I refused a port, despite having severe trypanophobia—an intense fear of needles—complicated by tiny, unreliable veins. My first infusion was administered through my ankle. The pain was unbearable. I had to be sedated.

From then on, every infusion required sedation. Panic alone felt terminal.

Eight months. Full-time work. Motherhood. Strength I wasn't sure I had.

Then, in the early hours of the morning, another call.

The cancer had returned.

Stage 3B metastatic melanoma.

And in that same call, I learned I was pregnant again.

The Cruelest Crossroads

I was told I could not carry the pregnancy. That my life was under immediate threat. That surgery to remove additional lymph nodes could not proceed while I was pregnant.

The timing was merciless.

It was the Jewish High Holy Days. I was at synagogue when my

OB-GYN called to say they would not perform a D&C. The ultrasound looked "fine." Ethically, they did not perform these procedures. They gave me the name of an abortion clinic instead.

It was 2:00 p.m. on a Friday.

I had planned to handle everything together—pregnancy termination and surgery—on Monday.

Now my husband and I were rushing to a clinic, my soul splintering in a waiting room I never imagined myself in.

That evening, my oncologist called again. A PET scan showed a lesion on my spine. I was told to go to the ER immediately for an MRI.

My first thought was simple and devastating: *If it's in my bones, I'm going to die.*

The MRI revealed a lesion that required biopsy. More waiting. More procedures.

Exhausted and hollow, we traveled to Colorado to visit my uncle—our first time away from our children. It was there, on his urging, that I met a man named Reuvain Bacal.

In two hours on a ranch, something shifted. Reuvain showed me how to quickly and effectively rewire my beliefs, my inner fears that were not serving me.

I left with hope. With clarity. With a willingness to choose life. With the understanding that cancer was not a death sentence.

I left feeling touched by God.

That moment became the foundation for everything that followed—my study of neuroscience, mindset, healing, and faith.

Chemo came next. It was brutal. My body could not tolerate it. After six weeks, we stopped.

In early 2018, I chose "watch and wait"—a medical phrase that deserves a gentler name.

I quit my job. I changed my diet. I was scanned relentlessly. My cousin Stephanie referred me to an incredible cancer coach, Leslie Kelly, who guided me through this journey. I was hesitant at first. I didn't want that kind of help. I eventually let go of the resistance that crept in and said, *I want to live, but I can't manage this alone.* Leslie was my saving grace. She offered me the tools, and I did a lot of mental and emotional work that led to significant shifts in all areas of my life—allowing me to live with authenticity and stop living for everyone else.

Eight years later, I remain NED—no evidence of disease.

The Identity Loss No One Warns You About

Cancer carries a silence no one prepares you for.
Not the silence of fear.
Not the silence of grief.
But the silence of losing yourself.
Protocols replace intuition. Numbers replace hope. In motherhood, you give pieces of yourself willingly. Cancer takes them without permission.
One day, I looked in the mirror and didn't recognize the woman staring back.
I was living—but I wasn't alive.
That terrified me more than cancer ever did.

The Return to Art

In 2018, I quit my job.
Not gracefully.
Not strategically.
But with a clarity that felt like oxygen.

I returned to art—the only language that had always known me.
Art held my grief when I had no words.
It held my trauma when I had no strength.
It held my dreams when I no longer believed I deserved them.
Canvas became confession. Color became courage.
Art stopped being my passion.
It became my purpose.
I acknowledge the privilege in that choice—made possible by my husband's financial support. Cancer carries an immense emotional and financial burden, one we don't speak about enough.

From Personal Healing to Collective Healing

My healing was never meant to end with me.
I began facilitating creative healing workshops—spaces for cancer patients, survivors, caregivers, adults, children—anyone who needed a place to breathe.
Art. Meditation. Writing. Movement. Neuroscience. Compassion.
Not therapy. Not "just art."
A bridge back to self.
Because stress can make you sick.
And creativity can help restore you.

The Truth Cancer Taught Me

Cancer was not my enemy.
Cancer was not my punishment.

Cancer was my teacher.
It cracked me open so I could finally see myself.
It turned pain into possibility.
Adversity into art.

Closing Reflection

If cancer taught me anything, it is this:
    Life is breathtakingly short.
    Joy is not a luxury—it is a responsibility.
    Cancer did not end my story.
    It revealed it.
    And if you are reading this—standing at your own crossroads—know this:
    Your story is not over.
    Your voice is not gone.
    You are allowed to become someone new.
    Sometimes your greatest challenge truly does awaken the opportunity to become your greatest gift.
    And you—
    you are allowed to receive it.

Nerissa's Grace Notes

- **Sometimes the wake-up call isn't gentle.**
  Cancer forced me to examine the parts of my life I ignored — and gave me the courage to change them.

- **The relationship you have with yourself sets the foundation for every other relationship in your life.** When you lose it, you lose everything. When you rebuild it, you regain everything.
- **Creativity is not decoration — it is medicine.** Art helped me heal when words and logic could not.
- **A crisis doesn't create truth — it reveals it.** Every fear, belief, and desire I had suppressed surfaced the moment life tested me. It's how I embraced it that saved me emotionally.
- **You don't have to choose between being strong and being soft.** Healing requires both.
- **Your body is not your enemy. It is your messenger.** Listen deeply. It always speaks truth.
- **Healing is not the absence of pain.** It is the presence of courage, compassion, and connection.
- **You are not obligated to return to the life you had before cancer.** That version of you is gone. You are allowed to become someone new.

Your greatest challenge may become your greatest gift.
    Not immediately.
    Not easily.
    But eventually, beautifully, and unmistakably.

The Art of Returning to Yourself
Alicia's Story

H*ow Alicia Reclaimed Her Body, Her Faith, and Her Future One Breath at a Time.*

What happens when life demands strength on a day you don't feel strong?
When your children still need breakfast, school drop-off, bedtime stories—
and you are the one suddenly fighting for your own life?
Alicia's story is a reminder that healing is not glamorous or linear.
It is raw, inconvenient, tender, stubborn, and holy.
It is the art of returning—again and again—to the truth
that you are worth fighting for.
Her journey invites us to believe in miracles both expected and unexpected,
and to trust that even after the darkest seasons,
something beautiful can still grow.

Nerissa Balland

. . .

The Shock That Split Her Life in Two

In 2013, at thirty-four years old—on April Fool's Day, of all days—
Alicia Palelis was told she had stage three breast cancer.
A mother of two young children, a devoted autism coach,
a wife with a steady rhythm of work, sports, playdates,
and a home full of movement—
cancer did not fit anywhere in her life.
And yet it arrived anyway.
She felt a sharp pain one day and reached for her breast instinctively.
A lump.
Her gynecologist said what many say to young women:
"You're probably fine, but let's check."
But the mammogram, the repeated images, the biopsy—
all whispered the truth her intuition already knew.
And then a nurse—trying to comfort—hugged her and said,
"Don't worry, you'll be around for your daughter's wedding."
A sentence that felt like a premonition.
Alicia left that room understanding there was no turning back.

Treatment Arrived Like a Storm

Her cancer was HER2-positive and already in her lymph nodes.
Everything moved fast:
a port placed within days, chemotherapy beginning immediately,
a double mastectomy, then radiation, then reconstruction.
Eleven lymph nodes removed.

She wore cold caps to preserve her hair—
not out of vanity, but for her students with autism
who might pull a wig and witness something traumatic.
Even while her body moved through trauma,
she worked hard to keep her emotional world upright
for her two young children.
She didn't use the word "cancer" at first—
not out of secrecy, but out of protection.
Still, her son put the pieces together,
and one day simply said,
"Everybody's getting cancer nowadays."
He knew.
He wasn't afraid. And somehow, that helped her breathe.
Her daughter, four at the time, became her "little doctor."
Showing up at radiation with coloring books,
passing chocolates to chemo patients,
helping nurses build a treasure box for other children—
transforming sterile spaces into places of tenderness.
Alicia learned quickly that community is not a luxury—
it is survival.

The Emotional Landscape No One Prepares You For

There were moments of deep darkness—
    especially after surgery, when the scars felt overwhelming
    and she whispered to her husband,
    "You picked the wrong one. I'm defective."
    Her husband and mother rotated caregiving
    so her kids' routines stayed intact.
    But Alicia still felt jealousy, guilt, and grief
    watching others take her children to activities

she used to manage herself.
She saw a counselor who gently named it:
"You are experiencing trauma. Healing isn't linear."
Target aisles made her cry—
just walking past shampoo she wasn't allowed to use
became a reminder of everything cancer had taken.
And yet, she kept moving.
Yoga. Journaling. Meditation. Art therapy.
Letting herself cry.
Letting friends show up.
Letting herself be held.
Slowly, the emotional waves began to soften.

Life After Cancer: A Return, a Rebirth

Alicia reached "no evidence of disease,"
but recovery wasn't the end of the story.
Fear lingered before every follow-up scan.
She deleted nearly 40 Instagram accounts
of young survivors who had passed away—
a digital graveyard she wasn't prepared to face.
But then something unexpected happened:
miracle disguised as biology.
Despite chemo's impact on fertility
and without medical intervention,
Alicia became pregnant—
two years after treatment, almost to the day her doctor said
"It's unlikely, but not impossible."
Matthew Hero was born in 2016—
her "cancer gift," her reminder
that life insists on blooming even after fire.

During her C-section, doctors removed her fallopian tubes
to reduce future ovarian cancer risk—
another layer of protection as she stepped into motherhood again.
Raising him now, she says colors feel brighter.
The world feels fuller.
She sees beauty more intensely.
She wears the good jewelry to Publix
because "Why wait?"
She understands time differently—
as something fragile, generous, mysterious.

The New Normal

Alicia still attends support groups,
still mentors young women newly diagnosed,
still reminds herself that self-care is not optional.
Her marriage is stronger—
bonded by storms weathered together.
Her relationship with her own body has healed slowly, imperfectly.
Her scars no longer tell a story of loss—
they tell a story of survival.
Her daughter now asks sometimes,
"Will I get breast cancer?"
Alicia answers honestly but gently:
"We don't know what the future holds.
But look how good Mommy is now.
If it ever happens, we'll get through it together."
Because that's what Alicia learned—
cancer may shake your life,
but it doesn't get to steal your power.

She reclaimed that power,
one breath, one prayer, one tiny act of courage at a time.

Closing Reflection

Alicia teaches us that healing is not a return to who you once were.
It is a becoming.
A becoming braver in the places you once felt fragile.
Softer where you once armored yourself.
Wiser in the knowing that fear may never fully disappear—but it does not get to lead.
Her story reminds us that life after cancer is not about reclaiming the old normal.
It is about learning how to live inside a new one—
one shaped by scars that no longer signify loss,
but survival.
Alicia learned to trust her breath again.
To trust her body, even after it betrayed her expectations.
To trust that joy could return—not loudly, not all at once,
but gently, like light finding its way back into a room.
She shows us that presence is an act of courage.
That wearing the good jewelry to the grocery store is not frivolous—
it is defiance.
That noticing color, laughter, and ordinary miracles
is how we resist letting fear shrink our lives.
Healing, she teaches, is holy work.
It is choosing to stay.
Choosing to love deeply even when loss is possible.
Choosing to believe that something beautiful can grow
from the very ground that once held devastation.

Alicia found her way back to herself—
one breath, one prayer, one small act of courage at a time.
And in doing so, she reminds us that returning to yourself
is not an ending.
It is the beginning.

Alicia's Grace Notes

- **You can acknowledge fear without living in fear.**
- **Let others help**—community is medicine.
- **You are not "defective"** because your body changed. You are alive.
- **Healing is nonlinear**—give yourself grace for the days that wobble.
- **Movement, mindfulness, and creativity are tools, not luxuries.**
- **Children can sense more than we expect;** honesty builds trust.
- **Your scars tell a story of survival, not loss.**
- **Miracles may arrive in forms you never imagined.**
- **Self-care is sacred**—it is your foundation, not an indulgence.
- **Life after cancer is not about going back. It's about becoming.**

The Art of Returning to Life
Christina's Story

F*rom dimpling and dread to hurricanes, healing, and the quiet miracle of a heartbeat beneath scarred skin—Christina's journey into reclaiming her body, her spirit, and her future.*

There's a particular kind of exhaustion that belongs only to young mothers: the bone-deep tired that comes from tiny feet at 3 a.m., sticky hands on your cheeks, and the never-ending loop of snacks, naps, and laundry.

Christina carried that ordinary tired—and then discovered it was hiding something else.

Her story sits at the intersection of so many layers:

- A family tree marked by breast cancer
- A body still nursing two babies
- A heart that leans holistic and spiritual
- A hurricane barreling toward Florida
- And later, a different storm—survivor's guilt—after losing a friend who didn't make it

Listening to her, what struck me most was how many times she had to choose: between holistic and Western medicine, between idealism and survival, between fierce independence and letting people literally keep her alive with crackers and sips of water.

And then—maybe the most radical choice of all—deciding to get pregnant again after cancer, not as denial, but as an act of faith in her own future.

A Midwife, a Dimple, and a Sentence That Changed Everything

In 2017, Christina was 37, living in Delray Beach with her partner and two very young kids:

- A one-and-a-half-year-old, still nursing
- A two-and-a-half-year-old, always in motion

She felt what she thought was mastitis: redness, firmness, a patch of irritated skin—classic clogged-duct territory. She called her midwife, the intuitive healer she trusted with her body and babies.

In the exam room, everything shifted.

Her midwife noticed something Christina had never heard of, even with a mom and grandmother who'd both had breast cancer: dimpling of the skin. The pores looked enlarged, the skin puckered in that one area.

And then came the words:

"I'm so sorry, but I think this might be breast cancer."

Christina was sent immediately for imaging. She was only 37—an age where mammograms aren't routinely covered. Thanks to her midwife's "call in a favor," she was scanned the same day.

The result:

- Stage III breast cancer
- HER2 positive
- Already in her lymph system

From "I think I have mastitis" to "You have stage three cancer" in a single day. With a toddler on her breast and a preschooler at home.

Holistic Heart, Western Medicine

Christina is, at her core, a holistic soul. Her first reaction in the oncologist's office—when they began listing chemo, port placement, surgery, radiation—was to laugh out loud.
"I'm not doing any of that."
It wasn't denial. It was shock—and a deep belief in the body's capacity to heal through food, plants, and energy.
So she pressed pause. For about a month, she went all-in on holistic protocols:

- Seven-day green juice fast
- Gerson-style nutrition
- Vitamin C drips
- Moringa from a local tree, ground fresh
- Oils, supplements, detox diets

She felt physically *amazing*—high on chlorophyll and discipline.
During that time, she leaned heavily on a new friend, Sarah, a young single mom in her neighborhood also diagnosed with stage three breast cancer. They traded tips, stories, and holistic ideas.
But as Christina experimented with juice and superfoods, Sarah's cancer progressed to stage four.
Her oncologist—a seasoned, 79-year-old HER2-positive specialist

who was part of the original Herceptin trials—held space for her holistic leanings but did not sugarcoat reality.

"You can keep doing your frankincense and vitamin C. I'll still be here. But I cannot guarantee you the same outcome if you come back in a month or two."

A nurse added a question that cut deeper than any statistic:

"How old are your kids?"

"One and a half and two and a half."

"Then you need to start treatment."

And then Sarah, now stage four, told her through tears:

"Don't wait. Don't do what I did. Start."

One morning, Christina woke up with her right armpit throbbing. She thought of her children, of the years she wanted with them, and made the decision:

She would do chemo. She would do surgery. She would do radiation. She would do *everything*.

Chemo, Hurricanes, and Mothering from Bed

The chemo plan was aggressive: six powerful infusions stretching from September to January. They weren't the "every three weeks, you get a small window of feeling semi-human" kind. These knocked her flat.

Side effects rolled in like waves:

- Blinding migraines
- Nausea
- Zero appetite
- Crushing fatigue

And then came Hurricane Irma.

Her first chemo treatment was followed three days later by the storm's landfall. She was:

- Newly infused with poison
- Vomiting
- Weak
- In a house *without power*

She didn't drink. She barely ate. For three days she spiraled into dehydration, her caregivers doing their best but not yet understanding how structured chemo care has to be.

Later, her oncologist would tell her she came dangerously close to needing emergency IV fluids in the ER.

This became one of her big realizations:

Good intentions are not enough; care has to be organized.

Somebody has to be the de facto nurse—logging medicine times, tracking fluids, prompting bites of crackers and sips of water.

Her mom flew down from New York and stayed for months. Her partner became full-time dad, caretaker, and provider.

Christina, meanwhile, disappeared into survival mode.

Her kids would tiptoe into the bedroom, kiss her, pat her arm, bring her water, then toddle back out. She missed them desperately, but her body was too wrecked to do more than exist.

She had to wean her nursing daughter almost overnight because of scans and toxic drugs. That immediate severing of a breastfeeding bond added another layer of heartbreak.

The emotional impact of all of it—fear, anger, grief—didn't fully land until halfway through chemo. The first months were a blur of chemical fog and migraines. Then, once she could think again, the rage hit.

High-dose steroids plus grief plus helplessness:

"I had never felt that kind of anger in my life. I was raging inside."

Knives, Scars, and the Radiation Room

After chemo, surgery.

She'd braced herself for a double mastectomy. But because of her breast size, her surgeons were able to do a partial mastectomy:

- They removed the entire right axillary lymph system
- Removed about half the right breast
- Reduced the left to match
- Reassigned nipples
- Left her three cup sizes smaller, but implant-free

Her right armpit is now permanently concave. Her arm numb, tingling like the lingering fuzz after a dental anesthetic.

Then came 32 sessions of radiation, laying her under the giant machine, skin slowly burning and tightening.

From diagnosis to finishing radiation, it was nearly a full year of continuous treatment.

Kids, Ports, and the Reality of "Honest But Gentle"

Christina and her partner made a decision early on: their kids would know the word *cancer*.

No elaborate euphemisms. No whispered secrets.

They told them things like:

- "Mommy has cancer."

- "This medicine makes me very sick, but it's helping my body."
- "The cancer isn't what's making me throw up—the chemo is."

The port in her chest was what frightened them most. They'd ask to look at it, fascinated and disturbed by the bump under her skin.

"Are you going to have that scar forever, Mom?"

Her daughter would tie scarves on her own head when Christina lost her hair. Her son called her bald head "silly." The kids adjusted in the way young children do: matter-of-factly, with an astounding ability to accept reality as it is.

Sarah, Stage Four, and the Heavy Weight of Surviving

As Christina crawled her way through chemo, surgery, and radiation, Sarah kept worsening. Stage three became stage four, and then the long, brutal decline.

Sarah was everything you'd put on a brochure for "doing everything right":

- Yoga instructor
- Spiritual teacher
- Holistic, active, vibrant

And still, her body could not be saved.

Christina watched her friend suffer unimaginably for two years. She watched her fight, even in hospice, cursing and insisting, "This is not going to fucking take me down."

And then it did.

After Christina was declared in remission, their paths diverged sharply:

- Christina grew stronger, went back to work, rebuilt her life
- Sarah's health crumbled
- Eventually, Sarah's daughter was adopted by another family member

This is where survivor's guilt settled in.

Christina wasn't ashamed of surviving. She was proud. But she felt a sharp, particular guilt:

- Guilt that she was getting better while Sarah was dying
- Guilt that their friendship changed when their realities no longer matched
- Guilt that she couldn't stay as close to Sarah's daughter as she'd hoped

She still stays in touch with Sarah's family. Her children still point to "magical" moments and say, "That was sweet Sarah."

Grief re-arranged itself into gratitude—but the guilt had to be walked through, not around.

Learning to Ask, Learning to Receive

One of Christina's biggest lessons wasn't medical—it was relational.

During that first chemo + hurricane week, she ended up dangerously dehydrated because no one realized she hadn't eaten or drunk anything for three days. Her caregivers were loving, but they were improvising.

She realized:

- Caregivers need direction
- She needed to say out loud: "I need you to bring me water every hour."
- They needed systems—lists, schedules, logs—not just vibes and hope

Another emotional minefield: the people who disappeared.

Some friends didn't visit. Some didn't text. Some mom friends never offered to take her kids for a playdate. Not because they didn't care, necessarily—but because they were scared, uncomfortable, or assumed she needed space.

When you are that sick, that silence can feel like abandonment. Christina's advice (born from hindsight, not perfection):

- Be honest about what you need from the people closest to you
- Let others know how they can help (meals, kid pick-ups, house cleaning)
- Recognize that caregivers also carry trauma and fear— and need appreciation too

Her partner later admitted how terrified and overwhelmed he'd been:

Responsible for finances, kids, household, and the emotional weight of possibly losing the person he loved.

Cancer didn't just test Christina. It tested every relationship around her.

Pregnant After Cancer: Choosing Life Again

. . .

About a year and a half after finishing treatment, Christina had several clean scans behind her.

But there was a ghost lingering: she'd had a miscarriage shortly before her breast cancer diagnosis. She had wanted a third child.

Now 40, she met with her doctors to understand her fertility. Tests suggested chemo hadn't fully shut down her reproductive capacity.

She and her partner had a choice:

- Play it safe and avoid pregnancy, out of fear
- Or try once more, fully aware it wasn't risk-free

They chose possibility.

It didn't happen instantly, but eventually, it did: two pink lines.

Now, as she tells her story, she's six months pregnant. This pregnancy feels different—scar tissue pulls, her post-surgical chest aches, and it remains to be seen whether she'll be able to breastfeed.

But she is clear about one thing: this baby is not denial. This baby is a declaration.

"It's a blessing to have survived and be brimming with life again."

Spiritual Practice and Letting Cancer Go

Christina still scans every six months. She still checks her body. She still knows what's at stake.

But she refuses to let fear be the main character.

She works with a practice she calls "power wishing"—a blend of affirmations, intention, and spiritual hygiene. Mantras like:

- "With grace and ease, I release any guilt for ever having cancer in my body."

- "My cells regenerate in health and harmony."

She knows it's not a magic force field. She still shows up for scans and follow-ups. But it changes the tone of her story—from bracing for impact to actively choosing life.

For a long time, cancer was the first thing she told people about herself.

"I'd find ways to slip it into conversation. 'Well, I had chemo last year...' I felt like I had to explain my haircut, my scars, my whole existence."

Now, she's letting the identity soften. She doesn't lead with it anymore. It's part of her, but not all of her.

Just like the port scar near her collarbone—it's there, permanent, but no longer defining.

Closing Reflection

Christina's journey started with a misdiagnosed "clogged duct" and landed in a chemo chair during a hurricane. It asked her to surrender control, accept help, and face the raw unfairness of watching a friend die from the same disease she survived.

And still—she chose to open her body to life again. To carry a child in a chest mapped with radiation burns and surgical scars. To braid gratitude into the ordinary days of preschool pickup, pregnancy aches, and bedtime stories.

Her story doesn't promise that everything will turn out okay. None of ours can.

But it does offer this:

We are allowed to change our minds.

We are allowed to ask for help.

We are allowed to survive.

And we are allowed, even after cancer, to dream in color about what comes next.

Christina's Grace Notes

- **Trust the intuitive people on your path.** Her midwife noticed dimpling and pushed for a mammogram that saved Christina's life.
- **Holistic vs. Western doesn't have to be a war.** She used green juice, herbs, and spiritual practices *alongside* chemo, surgery, and radiation—not instead of them.
- **Your caregivers need a game plan.** Write down:
  - Meds and times
  - Minimum hydration/food goals
  - Who's "on duty" each day
- **Say what you need—out loud.** "Come sit with me." "Bring me broth." "Can you take the kids for an hour?" People often *want* to help and just don't know how.
- **Expect some people to vanish.** It hurts—but it's often about their fear, not your worth. Focus on the ones who lean in.
- **Give caregivers grace, too.** They are scared and stretched. Your suffering doesn't cancel theirs.
- **Let the aftershock be real.** PTSD, chemo brain, rage, tears in the grocery store—they're not weakness, they're nervous-system realities.
- **Survivor's guilt doesn't mean you're ungrateful.** You can mourn the ones who died *and* be fiercely grateful you're still here. Both can exist.
- **Spiritual practice can be one of your medicines.** Mantras, prayer, visualization, breathwork

—none of these replace treatment, but they can radically shift your inner landscape.
- **You're allowed to build a future.** Having another baby, changing jobs, moving, making art—these aren't betrayals of your cancer story. They're the point.

The Art of Learning to Feel the Sun Again
Colleen's Story

She survived cancer, chaos, and an unkind marriage — and slowly, bravely, chose herself.

The call came while she stood in her kitchen, hand on the microwave, her nine-year-old son at her side.

"Colleen, it is cancer."

Time fractured. Her first thought wasn't medical—it was maternal:

I'm going to die. What about my kids?

Cancer didn't arrive in a peaceful life. It stormed into a home shaped by alcoholism, emotional volatility, and the constant pressure of raising two boys alone in every way except on paper. It entered at a moment when Colleen had already been surviving for years.

What she didn't yet know was this:

Cancer would not only take her into the darkest year of her life.

It would also give her the strength she needed to eventually walk out of a marriage that had been dimming her light for far too long.

Before the Lump

At 39, Colleen was raising two boys inside a home ruled by alcohol. She slept on the couch for safety. She managed school runs, meals, work, and emotional landmines—all while trying to shield her sons. Survival wasn't dramatic. It was daily.

Cancer didn't interrupt a peaceful chapter. It collided with an already breaking heart.

The Snow Day That Saved Her Life

On a snow day—because the universe sometimes intervenes—Colleen felt a sharp pain in her chest. She lifted her hand to rub the area and found a lump.

A same-day appointment.
A sonogram.
A biopsy.
A phone call in her kitchen.
Diagnosis: Invasive ductal carcinoma, HER2+ and estrogen-positive. Aggressive.
Within three weeks, she was scheduled for a double mastectomy.

The Doctor Who Gave Her Hope

Her breast surgeon at Stony Brook looked her in the eye and said:

"This is treatable. This is curable. We know how to fight it."

It was the first breath she'd taken since hearing the word *cancer*.

She went home and told her boys:

"I'll lose my hair. I'll be sick. But I'm not planning on going anywhere."

Inside she was terrified. But she decided fear would not be the only voice her children heard.

The Brutal Year

One year held more medical trauma than some people experience in a lifetime:

- Double mastectomy
- Six rounds of chemo
- Radiation
- Full hysterectomy
- Repeated infections
- PICC lines
- A sunken right breast
- TRAM flap reconstruction
- Endless appointments and exhaustion

The year stripped her body, her identity, her marriage, and her emotional bandwidth.

Still, she kept going.
Still, she kept mothering.
Still, she fought.

. . .

Cancer and Alcoholism Under One Roof

Her husband didn't go to treatments. Didn't hold her hand. Didn't offer comfort.
He used her cancer to gain sympathy—for himself.
He said cruel things no one should hear, especially not a woman fighting for her life.
The house suffocated her.
Her boys suffered.
But she stayed—for them.

A Village That Carried Her

And then something beautiful happened:
Her community rose up.

- Meals delivered
- House cleaned
- Fundraisers thrown
- Her kids' lacrosse team wearing pink
- Churches praying for her
- Family and neighbors filling every gap

They paid bills when her husband lost his job.
They kept her afloat when she could barely stand.
"The support was tremendous," she says. "It saved us."

The Bubble Era

. . .

When treatment ended, fear didn't.

She entered what she calls "the bubble"—a quiet, isolating place where she shut down emotionally. She stayed in her bedroom, or on a couch in her friend's house after leaving the marriage.

She didn't know who she was without cancer or chaos.

But healing has its timing.

Bit by bit, friends pulled her out:

Onto boats.

Into sunlight.

Back into laughter.

One day, standing at work, she lifted her face toward the window and felt the sun.

"I've never felt it like this before."

It was the moment she realized she was alive—and finally living.

The Fear That Never Fully Leaves

Years later, she found a lump in her armpit.

The fear was instant.

Her sons' fear was worse.

The biopsy was benign.

Relief washed over her—but so did the reminder that survivorship isn't a finish line.

It's a lifetime muscle you strengthen again and again.

Leaving to Save Herself and Her Children

It took 10 years cancer-free and a lifetime of emotional bruises before she finally left her marriage.

Her sons' voices made it clear:
If you stay, we're not coming home.
So she walked out.
Moved in with her best friend.
Started over.
And for the first time in her adult life, she was safe.
Now she has:

- A gentle boyfriend
- Grandchildren
- Adult sons who thrive
- A sense of worth slowly rising inside her

Is it perfect? No.
Is it hers? Yes.
And that matters more.

Closing Reflection

If you met Colleen today—the laughter, the grandkids on her hip, the woman who pauses to feel the sun on her face—you might never guess the storms she's survived.
But she carries them.
She carries the kitchen where the phone call came.
The chemo chair.
The PICC lines.
The couch she slept on to avoid her husband.
The bubble.
The fear.
The boys she fought for.
The community that held her.

The belief that God didn't give her cancer, but He walked with her through it.
She is stitched together with scars and sunlight.
And when she tells another woman,
You're going to be okay,
she is not promising perfection.
She is promising that—even in the darkest moments—there will be breath, and warmth, and help, and hope.
There will be a day when the sun touches your face
and you realize...
I'm still here.
I get to be here.
And that is enough reason to keep going.

Colleen's Grace Notes

- **Take it one step at a time.** Big pictures overwhelm. Small steps save you.
- **Don't compare your cancer to anyone else's.** Every "body" is different.
- **Accept help without guilt.** Your job is survival. Let people love you.
- **Talk to your kids honestly.** They fear what they don't understand.
- **Watch for signs of anxiety in your children.** Get support early. They carry more than you think.
- **Find another survivor.** Someone one step ahead can be your oxygen.
- **Notice tiny moments of gratitude.** Sunlight. Breeze. Laughter. Those are anchors.

- **Leaving a damaging home is also part of healing.** Your life is allowed to feel safe.
- **Faith can be medicine.** Even if all it grants is the feeling: *I am not alone.*

The Art of Holding On, One Step at a Time
Liz's Story

Some days courage is just a mother packing lunch, drying her tears, and walking her child to school anyway.

If Liz's story were a piece of art, it wouldn't be a bold mural announced to the world.

It would be a quiet piece of needlework: tiny, repetitive stitches made in the in-between spaces of life—after a 16-hour shift, between school drop-off and pick-up, in the hush of a chemo chair while the world keeps spinning.

Cancer forced her to pick up an invisible needle and start stitching a new pattern: one that holds exhaustion and gratitude in the same frame, that makes room for a little boy's fears and a daughter's devotion to her own father, that asks:

How do you keep showing up when your body is scarred, your heart is tired, and your child is clinging to you like you might disappear?

For Liz, the answer has never been glamorous. It's been simple, stubborn, everyday art: walking to the schoolyard, cooking dinner when she'd rather collapse, saying yes to another Uno game, and learning—slowly—to save a little thread for herself.

Before the Lump: Life in Motion

Before cancer, Liz's life was full throttle.

She was 39, working long, grinding days as a hospital clerk at Staten Island Hospital—often sixteen hours at a time. She'd graduated from nursing school but hadn't yet passed her boards, living in that in-between space of "almost" and "not yet." She and her husband had bought a house the year before. Stability, at least on paper, was finally within reach.

Most of her heart, though, lived in a small boy named Carlos.

He was six and a half when she was diagnosed, a classic mama's boy who had grown up with grandparents very much in the mix. When Carlos was only two and a half, Liz's father had been diagnosed with lung cancer. She became his driver, his chemo companion, his advocate. She sat through every infusion she could, rearranging work schedules so she could be there.

That experience carved a groove into her life: hospitals, oncology floors, waiting rooms. She knew what chemo looked like. She'd watched her father walk through it and stay alive. At the time, she was just a daughter. She didn't know she was studying for her own future.

By 2018, her father's cancer had stabilized. He wasn't "out of the woods," but life felt manageable again. Carlos was in school full-time. Work was steady. The worst felt like it might be behind them.

That's when Liz found the lump.

. . .

The Day Everything Tilted

In May 2018, she was scratching under her arm when her fingers caught something that didn't feel right—a lump, tucked near the lymph nodes.

Her doctor assured her it was "probably just an infected lymph node." Antibiotics, "don't worry," and the lump seemed to shrink. Life rushed back in. Shifts to cover, lunches to pack, homework to help with. She didn't push further. It's hard to demand more tests when the world expects you at work at 7 a.m.

Months passed.

In September, fresh out of the shower, she did a quick towel shimmy and caught sight of something strange on her breast in the mirror—a small spot that looked like a pimple, but deeper, not on the surface. Her inner alarm went off. This time she lay down and checked, again and again, hoping each exam would prove her wrong.

It didn't.

She called the doctor that same afternoon. Within weeks, she was swept into the familiar but now terrifying machine: mammograms, more imaging, biopsies. Because of her dense breast tissue, nothing about it was straightforward.

About a month after that first appointment, the words became official: stage 3B breast cancer, with multiple spots in the breast and a large cancerous lymph node. Later, genetic testing would reveal she was BRCA-positive as well.

She knew enough from her father's journey to understand: this was serious.

The treatment plan came fast and hard—chemo first, then a double mastectomy, lymph node removal, radiation, and finally a hysterectomy as risk-reduction because of her BRCA status. It sounded less like a treatment plan and more like a dismantling of the body she'd known for nearly 40 years.

Somewhere between the scan rooms and the consults, a new question began to haunt her:
How do I tell my son?

Telling Carlos — Cancer Through an Eight-Year-Old's Eyes

At first, she and her husband thought they wouldn't tell Carlos. They wanted to protect him, to shield his childhood from this new wave of fear.

But kids feel what we don't say.

He'd already watched his grandfather go through chemo. He knew what ports looked like and what "cancer" could mean. Only in his experience, Grandpa was still here. Grandpa's survival quietly laid a foundation of hope.

Liz realized he needed honesty more than he needed the illusion that everything was "normal."

They told him in simple, age-appropriate words: Mommy has cancer. The doctors are going to give her strong medicine to help. She'll lose her hair. She might feel sick. But she is fighting to be here with him.

At the beginning, he took it in with a kind of solemn acceptance. Grandpa had cancer and was still alive. Maybe Mommy would be too. He didn't yet understand the weight she was carrying.

That understanding came later.

Walking Through Treatment — One Step, One Scan, One Scar

. . .

Treatment unfolded like a harsh schedule she hadn't signed up for:

- Chemotherapy, with all its familiar names: the heavy hitters, the infusions, the fatigue.
- Double mastectomy with direct-to-implant reconstruction: her breasts removed, new ones built in their place—different, numb, painfully sensitive in ways her son couldn't understand when he flung himself across her chest to cuddle.
- Lymph node removal, including the large cancerous node.
- Radiation, with cumulative fatigue and skin changes.
- Hysterectomy, closing the chapter on ovarian risk and fertility in one stroke.

Her body became a map of incisions—on her chest, her belly, the quiet evidence of how hard she had fought to stay.

Carlos saw more than most children his age do: scars peeking out as she changed, fresh dressings, the new shape of her mother's body. He would walk in, catch a glimpse and say, in that blunt, honest way kids do, "Mommy, you have scars."

She already knew. But hearing it out loud always landed with a little sting.

At the same time, he watched her keep showing up.

There were chemo days when she crawled into bed, and there were others when she still made it to school pick-up, walked him home, and watched him play on the playground. She didn't always feel brave. Most days, she simply felt tired. But over and over, she chose the next step: the next infusion, the next early morning bloodwork, the next walk to school.

If her father's journey had once been her lesson, now she was the one unknowingly teaching Carlos what perseverance looks like: not glamorous, not Instagram-ready—just relentless.

. . .

When the Body Heals and the Mind Won't

By fall 2019, the major medical milestones were done.

She rang bells. She had her "last chemo," her "last radiation," her "last surgery" on the calendar. Her team told her they had "gotten everything" during surgery. Her scans and bloodwork did their quiet work behind the scenes.

But one sentence never came clearly enough:

"Right now, there is no evidence of disease."

Without those words explicitly spoken, her mind never found a place to land. She knew, intellectually, that the tumors were gone, the nodes removed, the hysterectomy complete. But emotionally, she stayed braced, like someone waiting for a second wave she couldn't see.

This is the invisible part of the healing phase no one warns you about.

On the outside, the world sees:

"You're done with treatment. That's amazing!"

On the inside, the questions get louder:

- *What if it comes back?*
- *What if this ache means something?*
- *What if I wake up one day and it's everywhere?*

Her days filled back up with work and parenting—early alarms, long commutes, 16-hour shifts, school runs, homework, dinner, laundry. Life looked "normal" again. But underneath, her nervous system was still living in the storm.

. . .

Carlos's Anxiety and the Weight of Being "The Safe Place"

Just as Liz's body began to heal, Carlos's anxiety began to surface more clearly.

At eight, he clung to her even more than he had at six. School drop-off turned into emotional tug-of-war:

"Mommy, I'm going to miss you."

"You'll see me in a few hours, baby."

"Yeah, but I'm going to *miss* you."

On her 16-hour days, he would unravel if she didn't call multiple times. If he was with her parents, her phone would light up: "He needs to talk to you." She'd duck out, step into a hallway, and talk him "off the ledge," reassuring him she was okay, that she was coming back.

He had watched her disappear into hospitals and operating rooms. Somewhere inside, a part of him was always watching to see if she might disappear again.

Liz became, simultaneously, the patient and the emotional anchor. Even on days when she felt like she was barely keeping herself together, she found words to soothe him:

"I'm here. I'm not going anywhere right now. I'm still fighting to be with you."

It was love in its rawest form—exhausting, holy, and heavy.

Support, Strain, and the Complicated Heart of Family

Liz did not walk this road alone.

Her father, now years into his own lung cancer story, showed up for her the way she had shown up for him. He drove her to treatments, sat by her during infusions, held space for the kinds of conversations only two people with matching scars can have.

Their relationship deepened. Illness, strangely, became common ground.

She also connected with women online who were walking through similar diagnoses—people who understood ports and pathology reports and scanxiety without needing the whole backstory. When she needed to vent, they were there.

Her marriage, though, became more complicated.

In the early months of treatment, her husband stepped in to cover school runs, household tasks, and the day-to-day care for Carlos when she couldn't. But as the year wore on—compounded by his own job instability and financial stress—he became quieter, more withdrawn. Less emotionally present just as her emotional needs became greater.

By the time treatment ended, they were still married, still under the same roof—but the relationship itself was frayed, thin in places that used to feel solid. It's an unresolved thread in her story, one she's still figuring out how—or whether—to repair.

Learning to Care for Herself (Without Permission)

Ask Liz how she copes, and she'll tell you she's still learning.

For now, her self-care is small and ordinary:

- Looking at pictures of Carlos when the fear rises, reminding herself what she's fighting for.
- Walking to pick him up from school when her joints will allow it, letting the rhythm of her steps calm her nervous system, even for ten minutes.
- Letting herself cry, scream, or yell when the pressure builds too high—instead of swallowing it down.

- Watching TV or zoning out when her body demands rest, even if the dishes sit in the sink a little longer.

She knows she needs more:
Professional support for Carlos.
Therapy for herself.
A creative outlet—like the cross-stitching she once loved—to give her hands something soothing to do while her mind recovers.

These aren't luxuries anymore; they're part of how she will rebuild.

Like a half-finished embroidery waiting in a basket, her healing is not done. But the pattern has begun.

Closing Reflection

Liz's story isn't wrapped in a bow.
Her marriage is still uncertain.
Her son's anxiety still flares.
Her own fear still spikes in the quiet hours.

And yet—every day she gets up, showers in the dark before dawn, drives to the hospital, or walks to the schoolyard. She checks homework, makes dinner, and sits through another Uno rematch because her son wants one more round.

This, too, is art.

Not the big gallery kind, but the kind made in kitchens and waiting rooms: small, repetitive acts of love that, over time, hold a whole family together.

Liz may not see it yet, but every time she takes one more step—back to work, to pick-up line, to her father's side, to the exam room to ask a hard question—she adds another stitch to the tapestry of her life.

The masterpiece she is creating is not perfect, but it is honest and fiercely human:

the art of holding on, one step, one scan, one small act of courage at a time.

Since the inception of this book and our first interview, Liz has continued to move forward with a strength that defies measure. She has faced profound loss—losing her father to lung cancer and her husband to brain cancer—yet she has not stopped choosing life. In her quiet, determined bravery, she studied, passed her boards, and became a nurse, pouring healing into others even as she learns, day by day, how to heal herself.

Her journey reminds us that resilience is not loud or linear. It is the steady, sacred work of returning to yourself—again and again—no matter what life asks you to carry.

Liz's Grace Notes

- **Take it *one* step at a time.** Don't try to swallow the entire treatment plan in one gulp. Focus on the next chemo, the next scan, the next post-op appointment. Survive in slices.
- **Let yourself feel awful when you feel awful.** On the bad days, be sick. Be sad. Be angry. You don't have to perform strength for anyone. Just don't stay trapped there—let the feeling move through and then take the next small step.
- **Ask your doctors for clarity.** You're allowed to say, "I need to hear this in plain language—right now, is there evidence of disease?" Sometimes the words *matter* as much as the labs.
- **Get support early—for you and your kids.** Find at least one person who "gets it"—a survivor, a friend, a

therapist, an online group. And if your child becomes clingy or anxious, it's not a failure to get them help; it's an act of love.

- **Don't underestimate tiny rituals.** A short walk, a few rows of cross-stitch, ten minutes coloring beside your child—these are not small things. They're your nervous system's reset buttons.
- **You are allowed to need help.** You were not meant to carry chemo, radiation, surgeries, parenting, work, and everyone else's emotions on your own shoulders. Asking for help is not weakness; it's survival

The Art of Showing Up
Jennifer's Story

How a young mom, a hard diagnosis, and a backyard sky turned survival into a shared mission.

There's a special kind of tired that comes with mothering young kids and chasing a career you've worked hard to build. It's the kind of tired you can still be proud of—full calendar, car snacks, a body that somehow keeps saying yes.

Jen's life, by her own words, was "humming along." Dream job. Two little ones. A body strong from yoga and lifting. Family nearby. On paper, it looked like the ideal set-up: full, noisy, purposeful.

Cancer didn't arrive as a dramatic collapse. It slipped in quietly— a strange vein, a smudge of color in the mirror after hot yoga, a feeling that something simply wasn't right. And from that moment on, "showing up" took on an entirely new meaning.

This is the art she's practicing now:

Showing up for her own body.

Showing up for her children in age-appropriate truth.

Showing up for other women who are, like she once was, trying to keep small humans alive while fighting for their own lives.

It began in a backyard, under a bright March sky, with a phone call that would rearrange everything.

When Life Was Humming

In late 2017, Jen was 34, freshly back in the flow after maternity leave. She was working her dream job as brand manager for a national coffee company, balancing creative strategy meetings with daycare pickups and bedtime routines.

Her body felt strong and capable. She lifted weights. Practiced hot yoga. Juggled long commutes and little-kid chaos. She had what many women in their thirties are told to want: a good job, a growing family, a life that looked "on track."

Nothing in her January physical hinted at what was coming. Her labs were fine. Her doctor was unconcerned. If anything, the worst moment that month was having the flu on her birthday—a bummer, but hardly a red flag.

Life, as she knew it, was still intact.

The Vein, the Discoloration, the Knowing

A few weeks later, Jen noticed an odd, prominent vein on her chest. Because she lifted weights, she dismissed it as a quirk of muscle and movement.

Then came the hot yoga class.

On a rare, indulgent afternoon to herself, she flowed, sweated, showered, and lingered in the quiet. Stepping out of the steam, she caught her reflection and saw a darkened patch of skin on her left breast—right where that strange vein had been.

She reached up. Felt around. And there it was: a lump she knew was not a clogged duct, not postpartum leftovers, not "nothing."

Her body had been whispering; now it was speaking plainly.

By the next morning, she'd made an appointment with her OB-GYN. When her husband asked if he should come, she surprised herself by saying yes. That alone told her something was different. She was not usually the "come with me to the doctor" type.

Her OB-GYN examined her, felt the lump, and didn't sugarcoat his concern. He fast-tracked her to a breast surgeon.

The next day was a blur of mammogram, ultrasound, and that sentence from the radiologist that lodged itself in her brain:

"I'm so glad you came in today."

Jen didn't ask why. She was too stunned, too suspended in the moment.

But she remembered it. And when she called her husband afterward, that was the sentence she repeated. It would echo in her mind long after the ultrasound gel was wiped away.

A Backyard, a Sky, and the Call

The biopsy followed quickly—breast and lymph node. At the end of that visit, her breast surgeon said the words that make time fold in on itself:

"I am 90% sure this will come back as a cancer diagnosis."

Jen drove home with those words pressed against her chest like a stone.

She went to work the next day, tried to focus, tried to breathe. But tears kept surfacing, uninvited. Instead of explaining herself to everyone, she quietly left, drove home, and lay down in the backyard.

The sky was clear, the light gentle. She took photos of the trees and clouds, almost instinctively. It was as if part of her already knew: *Remember this. This is the last moment before your life changes names.*

That afternoon, the surgeon called.

Her two little girls were inside the house.

Her body was outside under the sun.

The words "breast cancer" moved her formally from one life into another.

The subtype was HER2-positive, a protein mutation that makes cancer cells multiply rapidly. Further testing staged it at III—her tumor was about six centimeters, and cancer had already reached at least one lymph node.

Life wasn't humming anymore. It was roaring.

Chemo, the Party Corner, and a Community That Refused to Let Go

Treatment came hard and fast:

- A port placed in her chest.
- Six rounds of heavy chemo (taxotere and carboplatin).
- 18 rounds of Herceptin and Perjeta, targeted therapies to shut down HER2.
- A bilateral mastectomy with immediate reconstruction via expanders.
- 28 rounds of radiation, burning a tight grid of hope across her chest.

Her chemo days could have been solely about poison and fear. Instead, they became about people.

In the infusion room, Jen found what she jokingly called the "party corner"—a cluster of patients, including a man named Bob, who turned chemo days into something that felt a little less clinical and a little more human. They swapped stories. Teased nurses. Laughed louder than anyone expected cancer patients to laugh.

Behind the scenes, a different kind of network formed.

Jen grew up in Raleigh, surrounded by family and lifelong friends. When the diagnosis hit, offers of help flooded in—meals, childcare, errands, prayers, grocery runs. It was generous, beautiful, and completely overwhelming.

So she did something wise: she didn't try to manage it alone.

Her best friend, Michelle, became the "coordinator of everything"—the central node in a web of care. When people asked, *"What can we do?"* Jen could simply say, *"Talk to Michelle."*

Michelle organized:

- Meal trains – hot dinners and frozen food.
- Weekly grocery runs – basics for lunchboxes and breakfasts.
- A "call if she crashes" crew – nearby friends and family who knew that an evening phone call meant, *"Jen just hit the wall and Carl needs backup."*
- Laundry angels – a cousin who'd whisk away baskets of clothes and return them clean.
- Lawn care – relatives who stepped in so Jen's husband didn't have to juggle chemo, kids, and yard work.

For about six months, almost every practical need was held by the people around them.

Jen, who used to reflexively say "Oh, we're fine," learned a different muscle: receiving. Letting people show up. Letting herself be carried.

It didn't fix the nausea. It didn't erase the gut infection that knocked her flat near the end of chemo. But it meant she never had to face those days alone.

Motherhood in the Treatment Room

Jen's girls were three and one when she was diagnosed. Too young to understand staging and subtypes, but not too young to sense when something big was happening.

She and her husband decided on a simple framework: honesty without overwhelming detail.

They bought a children's book about a mom with breast cancer, one that described it as a "boo-boo you can't see" and explained that doctors would help fix it. They read it twice. Her eldest asked a few questions, then went back to being three.

Jen set clear boundaries with family:

You can acknowledge what's happening, but you may not unload your fear on my child.

She refused the label "sick."

In her words: *"I'm not sick. I've been given a diagnosis. We are treating that diagnosis."*

When it came time to shave her head, they made it a party. Close friends gathered. Her daughters watched as the clippers buzzed. At one point, her three-year-old squeezed her hand and softly asked, "Mommy, are you scared to cut your hair?"

"Yes," Jen said. "A little."

Her daughter held on through the first pass of the clippers. When she realized her mom was okay, she let go and went off to play, leaving Jen surrounded by adults who were struggling more with the moment than her own child.

The kids came to her head-shaving party. They came to her pre-chemo celebration. They were woven into the story, not shielded from it.

Months later, in a car ride, her now-five-year-old casually said, "Mommy, you had cancer. You had breast cancer."

No drama. Just a fact she'd absorbed from the conversations around her.

Jen and her husband had never sat her down to label it that way—but she'd been listening. Children usually are.

No Evidence, New Questions

In August 2018, after six rounds of chemo and a double mastectomy, pathology came back: no evidence of disease.

Jen's tumor had completely responded to treatment. Only the sentinel lymph node—the one known to be involved—was removed, and no further spread was detected.

It was the best possible news in a terrifying year.

Yet the hardest mental spiral didn't come with the diagnosis. It came after the "all clear."

About two months post-surgery, while in radiation, Jen developed relentless headaches. They were severe enough to trigger every fear: *It's in my brain. It's back. I'm going to die before my baby remembers my name.*

For roughly 24 hours, she lived in what she now calls a prolonged panic attack. This—this post-treatment terror—was the part no one had warned her about.

Her oncologist ordered a brain scan, which came back stable. The likely culprit was her body detoxing from months of chemo. But the rabbit hole was real, and she learned something critical:

Cancer is not just a physical event. It rearranges your relationship with mortality, your sense of safety, your nervous system.

Jen went back to counseling, this time to someone who had both nursing and therapeutic training. She joined online support groups, watched other women wrestle with scans, side effects, and "what ifs," and realized:

You are not crazy.

You are not alone.

And you do not have to white-knuckle this by yourself.

Work, Identity, and Rewriting "Busy"

Before cancer, Jen's identity was braided tightly with her work. She loved her job, her team, her role. Her worth and productivity were intertwined.

Chemo blurred that braid.

Her boss, to his credit, stepped in and took over her role so the team could keep moving. It was a practical decision—necessary and kind—but it also left Jen wondering who she was if she wasn't leading at full speed.

At home, everyone was doing everything for her. The freezer was full. The laundry got folded. Groceries appeared. She suddenly wasn't the doer in any arena.

When treatment ended, she realized she didn't want to go back to commuting 90 minutes a day, living on the margins of her kids' evenings. She left that role and moved into law full-time, joining a firm where she'd already been working of counsel.

Eventually, she carved another shift: keeping a part-time legal presence while stepping into a new role with the KL Cancer Fund as Director of Community Engagement—a job built around exactly what she'd been practicing: showing up, building networks, and connecting survivors.

And in her personal life, she rewrote her relationship with "busy."

Now:

- Evenings are mostly protected for family.
- She says no more often and more easily.
- Coffee or lunch dates replace after-work drinks and late dinners.

It's not that her life became suddenly empty or chill. She still works, mothers, leads, and dreams. But she's far more intentional about where her energy goes—and who gets her limited time.

From Patient to Connector

Out of her treatment year, Young Moms Against Cancer grew from a casual Facebook idea into a living, breathing network.

What began as five women in the Triangle area, all diagnosed with breast cancer while raising kids, evolved into a broader circle of young moms with all types of cancer. Partnering with the KL Cancer Fund, they raised money for research while also raising something less measurable but just as vital: visibility.

They made it clear that "cancer patient" doesn't always look like the stereotype. She might be the mom in the preschool pickup line, the one in yoga pants and a baseball cap, or the one standing in line at the grocery store with a port under her skin, trying to remember if they're out of milk.

As Jen steps into her role with the KL Cancer Fund, her work is to do on the outside what she was doing privately in chemo rooms and Facebook threads:

- Build survivor networks.
- Connect hospital systems with resources.
- Make sure young women with cancer know they are seen, supported, and not fringe cases.

Her law degree still matters. Her branding background still matters. But now they're woven into a mission that feels deeply aligned with the part of her that lay in the backyard under that March sky and whispered, *"If I survive this, I want it to count."*

Closing Reflection

Jen's story isn't about "staying strong" in the glossy, inspirational-poster sense. It's about learning how to show up—messy, scared, supported, and still willing.

She showed up for her biopsy, even when the radiologist's words made her stomach drop.

She showed up for chemo, sitting in the "party corner," IV pole and all.

She showed up for her daughters, letting them hold her hand while the clippers buzzed.

She showed up for herself in counseling, on quiet mornings with her journal, on afternoons when the anxiety roared louder than her optimism.

And now she's showing up for other women, building the kind of network she needed when she was 34 and terrified.

The art here isn't perfection.

It's presence.

It's the willingness to be honest about the fear and still choose connection, still choose community, still choose to keep your life open—just enough—for joy to slip back in.

For every mother who hears the words "You have cancer" and looks down at a toddler tugging her sleeve, Jen's story is a reminder:

You don't have to do this alone.

You don't have to be the hero and the project manager and the patient.

You are allowed to receive.

You are allowed to ask for help.

You are allowed to build something beautiful out of the hardest year of your life.

This is the art of showing up. Not once, but over and over, in big rooms and small moments, in infusion chairs and backyards, in board meetings and bedtime stories.

It's imperfect. It's holy. And it's enough.

Jen's Grace Notes

- **Delegate your care coordination.** Let one trusted person (like Jen's friend Michelle) manage meal trains, texts, and logistics so you don't have to.
- **Say yes when people offer real help.** Laundry, groceries, lawn care, kid pickup—these are not small things. Receiving them is not weakness; it's resourcefulness.
- **Include your kids, but filter the fear.** Simple language, honest answers, and age-appropriate frameworks ("a boo-boo you can't see") can give children security without overburdening them.
- **Guard your mental health as fiercely as your physical health.** Counseling, support groups, and medication (when needed) are tools, not signs of failure.
- **Don't underestimate the aftermath.** Anxiety and panic after "no evidence of disease" are common.

Needing help then is just as valid as needing help during chemo.

- **Know you can change your relationship with work.** A diagnosis can be a brutal reset button—but it can also give you permission to reclaim your time, your commute, and your boundaries.
- **Choose your words carefully with other survivors.** Remember that metastatic patients are reading the same threads. Encourage without implying that a stage or outcome is the only "good" one.
- **Ritualize the hard moments.** Turn head-shaving into a party. Invite the kids. Take pictures of the sky. Mark the days—the bittersweet, not just the milestones.
- **Let your story evolve into service, if and when you're ready.** You don't owe anyone advocacy. But if your heart nudges you toward mentoring, fundraising, or building community, trust that call.

The Art of Rising Again
Julia's Story

H*ow One Woman Learned to Grow Beyond What Tried to Break Her.*

Some stories of survival begin with a single moment.
Julia's began twice.
Leukemia interrupted her childhood before she even learned who she was. It returned again in adulthood, long after she believed that chapter was closed. But cancer was not the only adversary. Steroids, chronic illness, stigma, early menopause, depression, and questions about fertility became woven into the fabric of her life.
And yet — Julia speaks of her journey not with bitterness, but with a kind of grounded clarity earned only through deep emotional work. She learned to face her past, reorganize her future, and create meaning from what tried to destroy her.
This is the art of rising again — not once, but over and over.

. . .

A Childhood Interrupted

Julia was only eight years old in Caracas, Venezuela when leukemia first entered her life. The treatment was long and invasive — chemotherapy, endless medical specialists, isolated homebound schooling, and the disorienting experience of watching her childhood shrink down to hospital rooms.

When she was finally pronounced cancer-free, she grew into adolescence carrying both the weight of trauma and the desire to be "normal." But cancer had marked her early years in ways she didn't yet understand.

Peers ran from her, fearful that cancer was contagious. She felt like a monster — a young girl who learned too early to pretend she wasn't hurting. She played the brave one because she believed showing pain would hurt her parents more.

She buried everything and moved forward.

A Second Battle

At 40 years old, leukemia returned — suddenly and violently. This time, Venezuela didn't have the treatment she needed. Julia moved to Houston, Texas, where she underwent a bone marrow transplant from a non-related donor.

Her body rejected the donor cells.

Doctors fought back with high-dose steroids — life-saving, but toxic.

They saved her life, but they left permanent scars:

- Early menopause
- Cataracts in both eyes requiring lifelong monitoring

- Osteoarthritis and joint necrosis from years of steroid exposure
- And eventually, a severe depression that surfaced decades after she first learned to hide her feelings

Even after surviving cancer twice, it was chronic illness in her 30's that finally broke her open.

When the Body Breaks, the Emotions Surface

The diagnosis of osteoarthritis struck her harder than she expected. Pain, immobility, fear, and uncertainty collided with buried childhood memories — the stigma, the isolation, the pressure to be "strong," the guilt of never letting anyone see her cry.

Traumas she never processed came flooding back.

For the first time, Julia could not outrun her emotions. She couldn't stay busy enough, optimistic enough, or brave enough to silence them. She fell into a deep depression that forced her to stop everything — including the IVF treatment she and her husband were preparing to start.

It was the collapse that became her breakthrough.

Learning to Heal for Real

For most of her life, Julia powered through pain by staying in motion. School, work, responsibility, structure — all became anchors that kept her from drowning. But depression demanded stillness.

And in stillness, she finally had to face the truth:

Her body had survived, but her emotions hadn't healed.

So she began the slow work of rebuilding — through counseling, coaching certifications, psychological support, and learning to examine her life with new perceptual lenses. She learned to separate fact from fear, experience from identity, and story from truth.

Meditation helped her calm her nervous system.

Art — especially mandalas — softened her perfectionism.

Knowledge became a tool for self-discovery, not escape.

And her family, always her "rocks," became emotional ground instead of emotional responsibility.

For the first time, she let herself be held instead of having to be the brave one.

Facing Fertility, Hope, and the Future

Early menopause at 17 changed her reproductive landscape long before she knew what she wanted. She never produced viable eggs, but her uterus remained healthy — opening the possibility of pregnancy with an egg donor.

With honesty and courage, she explored IVF clinics across Venezuela, Panama, the Netherlands, and the U.S., navigating both the hope and the commercial chaos of fertility treatment.

When her osteoarthritis diagnosis disrupted everything, she put IVF on pause — not out of defeat, but out of wisdom.

She learned to ask a powerful question:

"Is my body ready to carry a child, and am I emotionally ready to be a mother?"

That clarity became its own form of empowerment.

Closing Reflection

. . .

Cancer gave Julia something she could not have gained anywhere else:

Resilience.

A deep, quiet bravery.

The knowing that she is unstoppable, but also allowed to rest.

It gave her a new purpose: to help others move through chronic illness, emotional trauma, and fear with compassion and practical tools.

She now supports people facing diagnoses, bone-marrow transplants, and chronic conditions — offering them what she needed most as a child and adolescent: a safe space to feel without judgment.

Cancer didn't just shape her.

It refined her.

It revealed her purpose.

Julia's Grace Points

- **You can survive something twice** and still learn the lessons years later.
- **Emotional healing often begins when the body finally collapses.**
- **Resilience is not the absence of pain** — it's the willingness to return to yourself again and again.
- **Support systems are not signs of weakness**; they are the bones that hold us up when our own body cannot.
- **Perspective, mindset, and knowledge are as therapeutic as medicine.**
- **You are allowed to redefine bravery** at every stage of your life.
- **Cancer may shape your path, but it does not get to write your story.**

The Art of Rising in the Ruins
Keilymar's Story

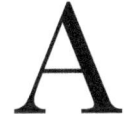 *young mother's journey through cancer, earthquakes, and rebirth — choosing resilience, faith, and self-care as her medicine.*

By the time I spoke with Keilymar, she had already lived through more upheaval in a few months than many people face in a decade: a sudden cancer diagnosis, a double mastectomy, earthquakes that took her home, a move from Puerto Rico to Connecticut, a pandemic, and the ache of leaving her little girl behind so she could chase treatment in another country.

And yet, what comes through most in her voice is not despair. It's steadiness.

She talks about science and faith in the same breath, about blessings in disguise and chemotherapy as a path to life. She describes losing her house and simply says, "The house wasn't my home. My home is where my partner is, where my son is, where my daughter is." She cries more over weaning her son than over the word cancer.

Listening to Keilymar, I was struck by how many times life had already tested her before the black mark appeared under her breast. A partner going to jail. Hurricane María. Fifteen flights of stairs while five months pregnant. Watching her daughter fall into depression and climb back out. It's not that cancer didn't shake her; it's that she'd already learned what she does when the ground moves:

She rises.

Her story is not just about surviving a diagnosis. It's about rebuilding a life while the earth, the healthcare system, and even her own body are all shifting at once—and still choosing to create something beautiful in the middle of all that rubble.

The Black Mark

At 28, Keilymar was in her last year of nursing school in Puerto Rico.

Her days were full and ordinary in the best possible way: lectures, clinicals, waitressing shifts, pumping breast milk between tables, and coming home to her children—a six-and-a-half-year-old daughter and a one-year-old son who was still very attached to breastfeeding.

Her breasts weren't abstract body parts. They were central to her daily life: milk, comfort, bonding, late-night feeds, pumping in the back of a restaurant. So when her partner pointed out a dark spot under her breast—"What do you have there?"—she looked.

It was a black mark, like a bruise, as if someone had punched her.

She hadn't been hurt. Milk was still flowing normally. But the mark didn't sit right in her spirit.

She called her doctor. He ordered tests.

On December 17, 2019, right before Christmas, she was told she had mucinous carcinoma, a type of breast cancer.

And then the world went quiet.

Clinics closed for the holidays. Doctors went on vacation. She had the diagnosis, but not the next steps. Everything paused, except her fear and her imagination.

When the Ground Literally Moves

Just as the new year began, the island shook.

On December 27, Puerto Rico was hit by a major earthquake. On January 6, more quakes followed. The hospital itself was literally trembling every half hour. Her surgeon didn't want to schedule a mastectomy in a building that wouldn't stay still; it wasn't safe.

At the same time, the earthquake damaged her home.

She and her family moved in with her partner's parents.

The timing was brutal:

- A new cancer diagnosis
- No clear treatment plan yet
- Hospitals that couldn't guarantee structural safety
- A first-grader who needed school
- A baby still nursing

So on January 17, 2020, she made an impossible choice:

She left Puerto Rico and moved to Connecticut with her partner and their toddler son, searching for stability and treatment.

Her six-year-old daughter stayed in Puerto Rico with her grandmother so she could finish the school year and have some semblance of normalcy. The plan was to bring her to the mainland when the school year ended and travel was safer.

That meant Keilymar walked into her mastectomy without her daughter physically near her.

In March 2020, at a breast specialty hospital in Connecticut, she had a double mastectomy with expanders placed. She chose both sides, even though the cancer was only in one breast, because she couldn't imagine living with one C-cup and one flat side—emotionally or aesthetically. She also wanted to reduce the chance of being dragged back into this fight again and again, like some of her relatives.

Surgeons removed a 6.4 cm invasive tumor. Mucinous carcinoma is often slower-growing, but in her case it had behaved aggressively. Based on the pathology, radiation, which initially wasn't expected, was now part of the plan.

She woke up flat, bandaged, with drains hanging from her chest and a body that would never be quite the same.

Nurse, Mother, Patient

Cancer wasn't the first time medicine had been in her life.

As a nursing student, Keilymar understood pathology, staging, chemotherapy protocols, side effects. She knew how to read a lab result and what a 6.4 cm tumor meant. That knowledge could have easily become fuel for anxiety—but for her, it became an anchor.

"I trust science," she says plainly.

She believes in God *and* in medicine. In her mind, they are partners, not opposites. Faith protects her spirit; the treatment plan protects her body.

That doesn't mean it didn't hurt.

The most devastating part at first wasn't hearing the word "cancer." It was the abrupt end of breastfeeding.

Her one-year-old son was still mostly breastfed, with food as the extra, not the other way around. When she had to stop nursing quickly to prepare for imaging, surgery, and treatment, he didn't understand. He reached for her shirt, tried to latch, and when she said no, he cried and lashed out—punching, kicking, pushing away from her. He started waking at night again, screaming.

"I think that hurt more than the cancer news," she admits.

After surgery, with strict rules not to lift him and fear that his little hands or feet could hit her incisions, she couldn't hold him the way she wanted to. She tried to bridge the gap with coloring, playing on the floor, and finding gentle ways to connect that protected her chest.

With her daughter, the conversation was different.

Because their family had seen cancer before, her older child already knew the word. Keilymar reminded her of relatives who had survived, like the aunt on her mother's side who'd had cancer three times, first at age 29, just a year older than she is now.

She framed her hair loss as something they could face together:

- "I'll probably lose my hair."
- "You're going to help me find the coolest hats and wigs."
- "You can help me with my makeup."
- "You can even do henna on my head."

At the same time, the life she had been building—finishing nursing school, stepping into a job at a clinic that was already waiting for her—was suddenly on hold.

Last year her world was about graduating and starting her career. This year, it's simpler and heavier:

"I just want to survive this so I can be there for my kids," she says.

Self Care by Kate

Because she's a visual person, one of the first things Keilymar did after hearing the word *mastectomy* was search for images.

She turned to Google, hoping to see real bodies like hers: young, recently postpartum, nursing, scarred, healing. Instead, she mostly found polished magazine spreads, older women, posed photos, airbrushed scars.

She didn't see herself.

So she decided to create what she couldn't find.

She launched "Self Care by Kate" on Instagram and Facebook—a space to show unfiltered glimpses of life as a 28-year-old mom in active breast cancer treatment:

- Photos of her post-mastectomy chest and drains
- Honest posts about pain, body image, and motherhood
- Reflections on faith, mindset, and her nursing knowledge
- Invitations for others to share their truths and images

Her best friend shared the page in online cancer groups, and women started to find her—some from the U.S., many Spanish-speaking women from Mexico, Peru, and other countries where the medical protocols and restrictions were surprisingly different. One woman casually mentioned swimming in the pool with her drains; Keilymar's surgeon in Connecticut had been absolutely firm: *no showers with drains, keep them bone-dry.* Even these differences became part of what she was learning and sharing.

At the same time, far from home and in a small borrowed room in Connecticut, she began returning to another part of herself: her art.

Before nursing school, kids, and double shifts, she loved painting and calligraphy. Life's grind had shoved that aside. In Connecticut, with no furniture of her own and long stretches of uncertainty, she ordered watercolors, brushes, and paper online.

She spread them out and started drawing, painting, lettering words.

Hours passed without her phone.

Art became her way to:

- Quiet her mind

- Get out of the constant scroll of cancer information
- Remember that she was more than a diagnosis and more than a body in recovery

She still loves yoga, and she dreams of a world where integrative medicine—yoga, art, mind-body practices—is covered by insurance and offered *as part* of cancer care, not as a luxury. For now, with limited upper-body range after surgery, she focuses on gentle lower-body stretches, breath, and brushstrokes.

She's planning to bring her sketchbook and paints to chemo, turning at least some infusion hours into a small studio, when her body allows.

Corona, Chemo, and Choosing Her Mindset

As if everything else weren't enough, chemotherapy for stage III breast cancer is starting in the middle of the COVID-19 pandemic.

Her original oncology hospital treated both cancer and non-cancer patients—too much risk for someone about to be immunosuppressed. So Keilymar advocated for herself and moved her treatment to a smaller clinic focused only on oncology patients.

Her plan:

- Stage III mucinous carcinoma with a 6.4 cm tumor
- Double mastectomy with expanders placed
- Chemotherapy: 16 infusions total
    - 4 treatments every two weeks
    - Then 12 weekly treatments
- Radiation afterward, since the tumor had been more aggressive than expected

She describes coronavirus as "the worst timing ever to get chemotherapy."

At the same time, she recognizes that this strange global pause has given her a few unexpected gifts:

- Her partner is home and can be fully present with their son because work is shut down.
- Life has slowed down enough to show her what truly matters.
- The move to a smaller clinic may offer more attentive care and less exposure risk.

Last year, everything in her world revolved around graduating, getting the nursing job, moving ahead. Now the priorities are stripped down:

- Survive treatment.
- Protect her kids.
- Stay emotionally and spiritually grounded.

She talks often about mindset:

"The mind controls so much. I believe the mind can even influence the cancer. If you go into treatment thinking, 'This won't work, I'm going to die anyway,' you're closed to healing."

She's realistic—she listens to her oncologist, understands side effects, and knows the physical battle ahead—but she also refuses to hand the rest of her life over to fear.

What she *can't* control:

- Genetics
- Earthquakes
- A pandemic
- The fact that her aunt had cancer three times

- Whether her daughter might one day face breast cancer

What she *can* control:

- How she shows up today
- The way she talks to her children about struggle and resilience
- The energy she brings into her own body and home

"I can't promise my daughter she won't get breast cancer," she says.

"But I can raise her with a mindset that helps her face whatever life throws at her."

Closing Reflection

Much of Keilymar's journey unfolds against a backdrop of instability: the literal shaking of earthquakes, the institutional chaos of hospitals balancing cancer care and coronavirus, the emotional tremors of leaving a daughter behind to chase treatment in another country, the tremble of a toddler's trust shaken by suddenly losing the breast that was his safe place.

And still, again and again, she chooses steadiness.

Not forced positivity. Not pretending everything is fine.

But a deep, practiced belief that even the darkest seasons can carry meaning, and that she has already walked through storms before.

She's seen blackness. She's seen her daughter's depression, her partner's incarceration, the wreckage of Hurricane María. She has learned, painfully, that life doesn't always go how we planned—and that sometimes the very thing that breaks you open also grows you into someone bigger, stronger, softer, and more present.

"The worst moments of my life," she reflects, "have given me some of my greatest blessings later. Maybe I needed to go through them to be where I am now."

The art of rising in the ruins is not about ignoring the ruins. It's about sitting in the dust of what collapsed—houses, plans, breasts, old identities—and choosing to build anyway:

- Choosing science and faith together.
- Choosing chemo and watercolor.
- Choosing to be honest with your kids and gentle with yourself.
- Choosing to see this not just as punishment, but as a doorway to becoming someone truer and more awake.

If there is a thread running through Keilymar's story, it's this:
You don't always choose what happens to you.
But you can choose how you show up—
and who you become on the other side.

Keilymar's Grace Notes

- **The black mark** under her breast—terrifying, but the warning signal that led to tests and likely saved her life.
- **Leaving Puerto Rico** not just because of cancer, but because the hospital itself was shaking in constant earthquakes.
- **The heartbreak of weaning**, and her toddler's anger and distance, teaching her that grief can look like kicking and screaming at 2 a.m.

- **Her aunt who survived cancer three times**, once at 29, becoming both a warning and a role model for fierce survival.
- **Cutting her waist-length hair**, donating it, and planning to shave the rest after her first chemo session, on her own terms.
- **Turning hair loss into a project** with her daughter —hats, wigs, henna crowns, and makeup instead of only loss.
- **Realizing her home isn't a building**, but the people she loves: "The house wasn't my home. My home is where my partner and kids are."
- **Creating "Self Care by Kate"**, turning her scars and drains into a resource for other young women who don't see themselves in polished stock photos.
- **The watercolors and calligraphy spread across the table**, reminding her that even in quarantine and chemo, she is still an artist, still a creator.

The Art of Carrying a Baby and a Diagnosis at the Same Time
Michelle's Story

L*earning to protect your child without abandoning yourself.*

There's a particular kind of terror when two realities collide: "I'm having a baby" and "I have cancer."

Pregnancy already comes with a thousand what-ifs. Add a diagnosis, and suddenly every decision feels like it carries the weight of two lives. Do I do the scan? The surgery? The chemo? What will this do to my baby? What will happen if I don't?

Michelle's story lives right in that collision—between medical necessity and maternal instinct, between privacy and needing help, between wanting to be "the strong one" and learning that strength also looks like saying, *"I'm scared,"* and *"I need support."*

Her journey is about:

- Navigating Hodgkin's lymphoma at 28 weeks pregnant

- Making excruciating treatment decisions while carrying her daughter, Ava
- Breastfeeding like a warrior on a deadline
- Cutting off toxic relationships, even when they were family
- Learning to honor fear without letting it run the show

And underneath all of it: the quiet, fierce truth that she wasn't just fighting cancer—she was fighting for the kind of mother, woman, and human she wanted to be.

Cancer in the Middle of "You're Having a Girl"

Michelle had just turned 28. She'd just announced to the world that she was pregnant and carrying a baby girl. Twenty-one weeks in, she finally shared the happy news. A week later, life tilted.

A lump appeared in her left supraclavicular area—just above her collarbone. Her doctor was concerned enough to move fast. Because needle biopsies often miss Hodgkin's, the surgeon recommended an excisional biopsy—cutting the whole lymph node out and sending it to pathology.

There was one big complication:

Michelle was 22 weeks pregnant.

Her general physician thought maybe it could be done under local anesthesia in the office. The surgeon took one look at the location—right by major arteries—and said absolutely not.

"If you hiccup or flinch, I could hit an artery."

So Michelle lay on an operating table, under general anesthesia, 22 weeks pregnant, while a mass was removed from her neck.

She remembers the consent talk clearly: spontaneous miscarriage was one of the listed risks. The surgery was necessary, but the guilt started there—before chemo, before staging, before the words were even official.

A week later, the pathology results came back:
Stage 1B Hodgkin's lymphoma.
23 weeks pregnant.

Two Doctors, Two Perspectives—and One Mother in the Middle

Michelle found herself between two specialists—and two different expectations.

Her oncologist said:

- Prognosis would not change if she delayed chemo briefly.
- If she chose not to do chemo during pregnancy, they could wait until after delivery, but he'd only give her about 2–3 weeks postpartum before starting treatment.

Her high-risk OB surprised her. Instead of focusing solely on the baby, he focused on her:

"You're not an incubator. You're a person."

He wanted to make *sure* delaying chemo wouldn't harm Michelle's long-term prognosis and was ready to advocate for treatment during pregnancy if needed.

Many people assume the OB will fight only for the baby, and the oncologist only for the patient. In Michelle's case, it was the opposite. The real tension landed on her shoulders: she had to live with whatever choice she made—for herself and for Ava.

She already felt the weight of that from the surgery:

"If anything ever goes wrong with her, I'll always wonder... was it because of that?"

She knew herself well enough to know: if she did chemo while pregnant and Ava ever got sick—or had trouble later in life—Michelle would carry that guilt like a boulder.

So, after weighing the risks and benefits, she chose to delay chemo until after Ava was born.

Ava's Birth and the Breastfeeding Marathon

Three months after her diagnosis, Michelle went into labor on her own. No scheduled induction, no C-section—just a vaginal delivery. Ava was premature, but here. Real. Tiny. Needing everything. And Michelle knew chemo was coming in about three weeks. That's when the mom guilt turned into mom determination. She knew premature babies benefit from breast milk, and she was laser-focused:

- Nurses and doctors gently told her, "You don't have to push this hard."
- They warned her about the pain of stopping milk production quickly.
- They reminded her she was about to start an intense chemo regimen.

She nodded.

Then she breastfed. And pumped. And pumped more.

"She was premature. She needs this."

By the time Ava was two weeks old, Michelle was producing around nine ounces every feed. When she finally had to stop to start chemo, Ava was able to live on Michelle's pumped milk for another full week.

Three weeks postpartum.
A newborn.
A body still healing from birth.
And then—it was time.

Chemo with a Newborn and No Pause Button

Michelle began ABVD chemotherapy: Adriamycin, Bleomycin, Vinblastine, Dacarbazine.

- Every two weeks
- 12 treatments total
- About 24 weeks of chemo

She described it simply:
"In the trenches, I thought I was just doing what I needed to do. Looking back, I don't know how I did that."

Her whole family—her parents, siblings—were in South Carolina.

Michelle, her husband, and Ava were in Ohio.

There was no village living in the next neighborhood over.

No revolving door of cousins and siblings popping in to help with the baby.

Her husband became the village.

- Up at 5 a.m. for work
- Full day on the job
- Home, straight into the shower
- Then: cooking, cleaning, baby duty

He was exhausted. She was exhausted. But he showed up, over and over.

"I don't know how he did what he did."

Michelle stayed home with Ava, trying to care for a newborn while:

- Recovering from surgery
- Recovering from birth
- Managing chemo side effects
- Navigating terrifying uncertainty

And somehow, in the middle of all that, she started to see people more clearly.

Losing Toxic Relationships and Choosing Herself

Cancer has a way of putting relationships under a microscope. Some get closer. Some fall apart. Some reveal truths you wish you'd never had to see.

Michelle had always been a "fixer"—the person who poured herself into broken people, overgave, absorbed drama, and stayed long after trust should have been withdrawn.

She also called herself a "doormat"—someone who gave endless chances, even when she knew she was being used.

During treatment, two major relationships fell away:

1. Her long-time best friend
    - Used Michelle's diagnosis as a sympathy magnet.
    - Social media posts about "my best friend with cancer" flowed constantly.

- But help? Showing up to hold the baby, clean a kitchen, sit with her during chemo? Her friend wasn't present.

Michelle realized: she was a story to this friend—a way to collect attention and praise online—more than a human being in need.
When she finally cut ties, people quietly came forward:
"We're really glad you finally cut her off. How did you not see how awful she was?"

2. Her sister. Without going into all the details, Michelle lost that relationship too. Painful, but clarifying.

What she gained instead was:

- A stronger marriage—a husband who backed her decisions and stood beside her in the worst moments.
- A smaller, more solid inner circle—people who saw her as *Michelle*, not just "the cancer friend."
- A new willingness to set boundaries and say, "No more."

The Long Tail: Fatigue, Triggers, and a Mind That Still Remembers

Today, Michelle is:

- In remission
- Out from diagnosis
- Living in South Carolina, now under the care of a new oncologist

Her scans are clear—but that doesn't mean the story is "over."
Cancer left fingerprints on her body:

- Chronic fatigue
- Sleep apnea (diagnosed after treatment)
- Hypothyroidism, adding another layer of exhaustion

Some days, she's just tired because: toddler + life.
Some days, she's tired and her brain whispers, *"Or is it back?"*
Her biggest triggers look like this:

- Night sweats: She originally wrote them off as normal pregnancy heat. Now, if she wakes up drenched, panic can spike.
- Nausea: A wave of queasiness and suddenly she's back in the chemo chair in her mind.
- Bone-deep fatigue: Hard to untangle from motherhood and other medical issues.

The old Michelle might have spiraled for 20, 30 minutes—or all night.
The current Michelle is learning a new practice.
"In the moment, cancer is always the #1 explanation. But then I walk it down the list."
Now when fear rises, she:

1. Acknowledges it
   - *"You have every right to be afraid. You've been through a lot."*
2. Looks for other explanations
   - It's hot. The AC was off.
   - Ava woke up twice last night.

- It's allergy season. You always feel off this time of year.
3. Moves cancer down the list
    - Instead of "it must be cancer,"
    - It becomes, *"Okay, maybe it's #5 on the list of possible reasons."*

She doesn't pretend she isn't scared.
She just doesn't let fear drive the car anymore.
And she uses healthy distraction too:

- Going on walks with Ava (when the weather cooperates).
- Coloring together—something that calms them both while giving them quality time.
- Crocheting (when her supplies aren't in storage).
- Reading (though sometimes the to-do list still tries to nag her out of it).

There's another tool she used that became deeply important:

Journaling: A Safe Place to Tell the Truth

During pregnancy and early treatment, Michelle kept a journal. In those pages, she:

- Poured out fear, anger, and grief without worrying how it sounded.
- Didn't have to reassure anyone else.
- Didn't have to hear, "You're so strong" when she felt anything but.

- Didn't worry about her emotions becoming someone else's drama.

It was just her, the pen, and the page.
Later, rereading that journal was unexpectedly powerful:
"It helped me see how far I'd come. What I was writing then, and where I am now—there's such a difference."
For someone private like Michelle, journaling gave her:

- A place to process.
- A record of her growth.
- A way to validate her own experience without needing external permission.

Closing Reflection

Michelle said something near the end of our conversation that stuck with me:
"When treatment ends, people think you're 'back to normal.' But they stayed on the main timeline. You dropped into a different one. You lived something they didn't. When you come back, you're not standing in the same place anymore."
If you're reading this while pregnant and newly diagnosed, or holding a baby with chemo on your calendar, you might feel exactly that:
like everyone else is on one track and you're on another—under the same sky, but in a different world.
Michelle's story doesn't pretend that world is easy.
It *does* show that:

- You can weigh your options and make decisions you can live with.
- You can love your child fiercely *and* still claim your right to be treated as a person, not just an incubator.
- You can lose people you thought you'd have forever—and still gain a stronger, more honest life.
- You can be terrified and still move forward, one small practice at a time.

You don't have to fix everything today.
Maybe today, you just:

- Write one raw page in a notebook.
- Ask one person for one specific kind of help.
- Color one page with your child.
- Remind yourself, *"Not every symptom is cancer. I'm allowed to consider other reasons, too."*

Healing—in your body and in your mind—isn't a switch that flips when chemo ends or when someone says the words "in remission."
It's a practice.
And like Michelle, you are allowed to take the time you need to learn it. In the six years since our first interview, Michelle has reconciled with her sister. She is cancer-free. And she has also endured the profound loss of her husband. Time is both fragile and exacting, and it reminds us that healing does not end when treatment stops or when we enter remission.

The skills you cultivate during your cancer journey—self-compassion, presence, resilience, and the courage to keep choosing yourself—are the very tools that will carry you through every adversity that follows. Surviving cancer is not a single chapter; it is a lifelong practice of showing up, again and again, for the life that is still unfolding.

Canvas of Courage

. . .

Michelle's Grace Notes

- **Letting herself make the final call**
    - On delaying chemo until after birth.
    - On which risks she could live with.
    - On cutting off toxic relationships.
    - Being "in control" of those decisions helped her live with them.
- **Asking for help (and wishing she'd asked for more).** She now wishes she had:
    - Asked someone to **coordinate support** (meals, laundry, baby help).
    - Assigned one trusted person to be the "point person" so she didn't have to manage logistics while in survival mode.
- **Finding at least one friend who saw her as more than a cancer patient.** A fellow new mom who treated her like a *person*, not just "my friend with cancer," made a huge difference.
- **Using journaling as a private place to be raw and honest.** A space where:
    - No one told her she was "overreacting".
    - No one said, "be positive".
    - She could admit, "I don't want to die," without editing herself.
- **Practicing fear reframe (over and over).**
    - Notice the trigger.
    - Name the fear.
    - List other, more likely explanations.
    - Move "cancer" down the list.
- **Choosing soothing, simple creative acts.**

- Coloring with Ava.
- Crocheting blankets and hats.
- Walks outside to move her body and shift her nervous system.

- **Accepting that recovery is not automatic.**

"It gets better—but not on its own. You have to participate in your own healing."

The Art of Being Held
Shauna's Story

L*earning to let go, lean in, and let love carry what you can't control.*

Motherhood often asks us to surrender—our sleep, our bodies, our time, our expectations. But cancer asks us to surrender differently. It strips away the illusion that we can control the unfolding of our lives. And yet, inside that unraveling, something else quietly rises: the courage to be held.

For many women, letting others carry the weight feels foreign, even wrong. We are conditioned to be strong, to keep going, to shoulder everything ourselves. Shauna's story is a tender reminder that sometimes the bravest thing a woman can do is soften into the arms that want to hold her.

Her journey—woven through infertility, new motherhood, a rare breast cancer diagnosis, and the terrifying unknowns of treatment—reveals a truth so many young mothers facing cancer feel but rarely speak:

It is not weakness to need help. It is humanity. And sometimes, it is survival.

Life Before Cancer: A Baby Hard-Fought and Deeply Loved

For seven long years, Shauna and her husband, Patrick, tried to conceive. Infertility carved deep emotional grooves into their marriage—physically exhausting, financially draining, and emotionally brutal. Through therapy, Shauna learned to replace the word *broken* with gentler language—crushed, wrinkled, worn. Something that could still be smoothed back into shape.

IVF finally brought them their daughter, Raegan. They moved for Patrick's dream job, Shauna changed careers for a more family-friendly role, and life was finally stitching itself together.

Then, at 36 weeks pregnant, she found a lump.

The Lump That Changed Everything

Her OB took her seriously—something many young mothers don't experience. After waiting one week, the ultrasound showed something suspicious. Due to the risk of triggering labor during a biopsy, they induced her at 39 weeks.

She gave birth to Raegan, breastfed with surprising success despite PCOS—and three days later, she lay on a biopsy table.

Her surgeon was nearly certain it was benign.

Four days postpartum, he called.

His voice gave everything away.

He'd refreshed the pathology page over and over, unwilling to believe it.

"I hate telling anyone they have breast cancer," he said. "And I especially hate telling a woman who delivered her daughter four days ago."

Shauna collapsed to the bedroom floor. Motherhood and cancer —two life-altering identities—arrived in the same week.

Choosing Control When Life Spun Out of It

Chaos pushed Shauna toward clarity.

She identified the few things she *could* control:

1. Her mental health

With postpartum hormones, a history of anxiety, and PCOS, she knew she needed medical and emotional support immediately.

2. Her daughter's safety

Would she breastfeed? Could she hold Raegan after chemo? What did motherhood look like now?

3. Who carried the emotional load

Shauna—a natural helper—forced herself to ask for help. She enlisted a point person, Blythe, to run communication, meal trains, and logistics.

4. Her information boundaries

She and Patrick made a pact not to Google anything until they heard directly from specialists. Afterward, they only researched credible medical sites.

5. The story she told

She journaled on PostHope so she didn't have to relive the trauma repeatedly. Her husband could update it on the days she couldn't.

This was how she stayed standing.

Treatment: Red Devil, Baking Days, and a New Kind of Motherhood

Shauna's staging: Stage II A–B
Her cancer was uniquely complex—borderline hormone-positive yet also treated as triple-negative.
Her oncology plan:

- 6 rounds of AC ("red devil")
- 12 rounds of Taxol
- Lumpectomy
- Double mastectomy
- Oral chemo (8 cycles of Xeloda)
- Long-term hormone therapy

She faced challenges unique to new mothers:

- She needed childcare for a newborn during each infusion.
- For 48 hours after chemo, she couldn't have Raegan directly against her skin—so she used a special blanket system to still hold her daughter.
- She mourned the loss of breastfeeding, especially after being told PCOS might make lactation impossible.

And still—she found her joy.
Baking became her self-care.
"The day before chemo, when I felt the best, I'd bake. Raspberry cream-cheese rolls, cupcakes from scratch. It was how I stayed me."

She brought the baked goods to nurses at every infusion. They were confused—but she wasn't:

"Baking was how I took my power back."

The Plan Falls Apart: A Rare Chemo Reaction

Midway through Taxol, her oxygen dropped dangerously low. She was hospitalized with Taxol-induced pneumonitis, a rare but severe reaction that can be fatal. Taxol was immediately stopped.

Suddenly, the plan changed:

- Lumpectomy first, since her lungs couldn't withstand long surgery
- Then months on oxygen
- Then double mastectomy
- Then Xeloda, which she tolerated better than expected

She also developed lymphedema—another rare complication.

Shauna joked often that she must be the "1% girl," collecting the side effects no one else got.

But then came the scare that shook her deeper than diagnosis.

The Shadow on Her Shoulder

Severe shoulder pain led to imaging. They saw a small suspicious lesion—possible metastasis.

Shauna and Patrick had some of the most painful "real talk" of their lives. They prepared themselves for bad news.

A bone scan came back clear, but the lesion was small enough to be missed.

A PET scan was ordered.

Shauna—normally private—went fully public and asked for prayers.

And then the phone rang again:

The PET scan was completely negative.

No cancer.

No spread.

No evidence of disease.

Ironically, she would never have received full-body imaging without that shoulder pain.

"It was terrifying, but it gave me a gift—confirmation I wasn't expecting."

Faith, Donor Milk, and the Quiet Places Where Hope Lives

Shauna didn't spend much time in church buildings during treatment, but faith still lived in her home—in quiet, consistent ways.

Every night during feedings or pumping, she read devotionals on the Bible App—breast cancer devotions, new mom devotions, healing scriptures.

Her faith wasn't loud; it was steady.

She also accepted help in a form many new mothers never consider:

Donor breast milk.

Friends—and later strangers—supplied breast milk vetted by her pediatrician's lactation consultant. Raegan received breast milk for her entire first year.

Other organizations stepped in:

- The Helene Foundation provided bi-weekly house cleaning and freezer meals for six months.
- Young Moms Against Cancer connected her with women who understood her world.
- Kick-Ass Cancer Moms, for women diagnosed during pregnancy or postpartum, gave her emotional grounding she couldn't find elsewhere.

She also made a painful but necessary self-care decision: sending Raegan to daycare so she could sleep between oral chemo cycles.

"It made me feel like a bad mom. But other cancer moms said, 'This is how you survive. This is how you mother.'"

They were right.

Closing Reflection

Shauna's journey reminds us that resilience is not the ability to push through alone—it is the willingness to be supported. The art of being held is a quiet, powerful form of courage that emerges when everything else has been stripped away.

Her story asks us to reconsider what strength looks like. Sometimes it is shaved heads and scarred chests. Sometimes it is whispered prayers at 3 a.m. Sometimes it is a woman handing her baby to someone else so she can sleep. Sometimes it is letting a friend organize a meal train, accepting a stranger's breast milk, or telling the truth in a "real talk" moment with a spouse.

Healing is rarely linear. But in the hands that hold us, the communities that circle us, and the faith that steadies us, we find the shape of a new life—one built not on perfection, but on presence.

Shauna's new normal is not what she imagined. But it is hers.

And she is here—awake, alive, held—and learning that sometimes the softest place we land becomes the strongest place we rise from.

Shauna's Grace Notes

- **You are not broken.** Infertility, IVF, body changes, and cancer don't diminish your worth.
- **Asking for help is wisdom, not weakness.** A point person can save your sanity—and your energy.
- **Control what you can and release the rest.**
  - Control: journaling, appointments, routines, boundaries.
  - Not in your control: diagnoses, timelines, other people's reactions.
- **Your mental and emotional health *are* part of treatment.**
- **Your baby will be okay—and so will you.** A mother who rests is a mother who stays.
- **Let people hold you.** This is not a journey for one set of hands.

The Art of Trusting Your Inner Voice
Chelsea's Story

*S*ometimes the body whispers the truth long before the world is ready to believe it.

When I think of Chelsea, I think of a woman who *technically* "did everything right" and still got knocked off her feet—and then chose to stand even taller. She grew up with cancer woven into her family story: a mom who faced breast cancer three times, a grandmother with breast and colon cancer, multiple relatives lost to the disease, and the BRCA gene running through the family tree.

At 30, she made what felt like the bravest, smartest, most proactive decision she could: a preventative double mastectomy, determined to save her own life before cancer ever had the chance.

And then, in the middle of doing the "right" thing, came the sucker punch: pathology revealing a tiny, aggressive tumor hidden in breast tissue that had already been removed. No lump she missed. No screening she skipped. Just a reminder that sometimes cancer doesn't follow the rules.

Chelsea's story holds a special kind of grief and power—grief for the illusion of control we all want so badly, and power in the way she trusted herself anyway. She listened to her gut when others told her a double mastectomy was "too drastic." She honored her future by freezing eggs before chemo. She let go of friendships that were draining, opened herself to the quiet love that had been in front of her for years, and later chose her happiness over a toxic work culture—even if that meant stepping "backward" on paper.

If you're reading this and wrestling with big decisions, second-guessing yourself under the weight of everyone's opinions, Chelsea's story is a reminder that your intuition about *your* body and *your* life is not only valid—it might just be life-saving.

Growing Up in the Shadow of Cancer

By the time Chelsea reached her twenties, cancer wasn't an abstract fear or a story about someone's "friend of a friend." It lived in her family.

Her mom was a three-time breast cancer survivor.

Her grandmother had survived breast and colon cancer.

Her mom had also buried her father and both brothers because of cancer.

Cancer had its own seat at every family table, every holiday, every whispered conversation in hallways.

When Chelsea's gynecologist was updating her medical history and casually asked, *"Does your mom have the BRCA gene?"* she honestly didn't know. She called her mom afterward—and got her first shock.

Her mom did have BRCA1, but had been told *not* to tell her daughters until they turned 27. At the time of her first diagnosis, doctors advised:

"Tell your daughters ten years before the age you were when you were diagnosed."

Her mom was 37 at diagnosis, so 27 became the magic number.

But Chelsea and her twin sister were 23.

And the reality was clear:

- People were being diagnosed younger and younger.
- Cancer had already knocked on their door—several times.

So instead of waiting, they decided to know.

They got tested.

Chelsea tested positive for BRCA1.

Her twin sister did not.

That result brought its own complicated mix of emotions—gratitude, fear, relief, guilt, and an invisible line drawn between two sisters who had shared everything since birth.

But more than anything, Chelsea felt this:

"If I know, I can do something."

And that became a turning point.

Living With the BRCA Gene: A Life of Surveillance

Knowing she carried the gene didn't mean she got cancer.

It meant she lived with a ticking clock and a permanent "high-risk" label.

From age 25, Chelsea entered a new rhythm:

- Annual MRIs
- Ultrasounds and mammograms
- Screenings every six months

She built a relationship with her oncologist long before she ever became "a patient with cancer." Her doctor knew her family, her fears, her questions.

And eventually, that same oncologist gently raised a possibility:

"When you turn 30, I want you to start *thinking* about a preventative double mastectomy."

Not a command.

Not a deadline.

A door, left open.

There were factors to consider:

- She didn't have children yet.
- Breastfeeding might or might not matter to her.
- Surgery is permanent—and visible.

But just as there is generational trauma, there is also generational wisdom. Chelsea had watched her mother walk this road three times. She had seen what cancer could take.

Deep down, she carried a quiet certainty:

"I always knew I would get cancer one day."

That belief didn't make her fatalistic.

It made her decisive.

At 29, she made up her mind:

When she turned 30, she would have a preventative double mastectomy.

She was single.

She wasn't attached to the idea of breastfeeding.

She wanted her future more than she wanted her original breasts.

So she spent a year doing what many people never see behind-the-scenes:

- Meeting multiple surgeons.
- Researching options.

- Sitting in consult rooms with her mom.
- Asking hard questions about reconstruction, scars, recovery, and risk.

By the time her 30th birthday came, she wasn't flippant or impulsive.

She was prepared.

The Party Before the Storm

Most people imagine pre-surgery days as somber and heavy. Chelsea chose something very different.

For her 30th birthday, she went to Mexico with seven of her closest friends.

On the beach, they did a naked photo shoot—a farewell to the body she'd had for three decades, and a celebration of the body that had carried her this far.

Those photos weren't about vanity.

They were about agency.

"I was saving my own life. This was something I was choosing, not something being done to me."

She walked into surgery two weeks later already having said goodbye.

On July 16, 2018, just after her 30th birthday, Chelsea had her preventative double mastectomy.

Her surgeons removed her breast tissue.

They sent it, like they always do, to pathology.

And everyone expected the final report to say what they all believed to be true:

Benign. Clear. Preventative.

But cancer doesn't always cooperate with our plans.

"We Found Cancer": When Preventative Became Real

A week after surgery, Chelsea was at her mom's house, recovering.

Her mom had gone back to work for the first time.

Her mom's best friend was with her, keeping an eye on her, helping her manage drains and pain medication.

The phone rang.

It was her doctor.

She put it on speaker.

The voice on the other end sounded calm, almost casual—the way doctors often sound when they've practiced saying hard things.

"Your left breast came back totally clean."

"But we did find cancer in your right breast."

Just like that.

In one breath, Chelsea's surgery shifted from preventative to treatment.

It wasn't a hypothetical anymore.

There was a tumor—

- Triple negative
- About 7 millimeters
- So small it might have been missed by a less meticulous pathologist

Three months earlier, her MRI had shown nothing.

By the time of surgery, a fast-growing tumor was already there.

Her doctor continued:

- She'd need another surgery to remove lymph nodes.
- They needed to make sure nothing had spread.

- Chemo would now be part of the plan—not optional, not theoretical, but real.

Chelsea remembers sitting there, in shock, with her mom's best friend and her stepdad, all three of them wide-eyed, trying to absorb too much information too fast.

And then another dread crept in:

"How do I tell my mom?"

Her mom had just gone back to work. She thought the hardest part was over.

They decided to wait.

Chelsea spent the day feeling sick with anxiety, stomach in knots, mind racing.

When the garage door finally opened that afternoon, everyone tensed.

Her mom walked in.

Took one look at their faces.

And knew.

"What's wrong?"

Chelsea told her.

Her mom's eyes filled with tears—but she didn't crumble.

"All right. We'll do this. We've got this."

Her mom had been through cancer three times. She knew what it meant—and what it didn't have to mean. That steadiness became one of Chelsea's anchors.

Fertility, Chemo, and Rewriting the Timeline

Once the diagnosis became official, everything sped up.

Even though the tumor was small and caught early, it was triple negative, which tends to be more aggressive and has fewer targeted treatment options.

The recommendation: chemotherapy, not just to treat what had been found, but to reduce the risk of anything lingering in her blood or hiding somewhere else.

Chelsea had to juggle questions that most 30-year-olds never imagine asking themselves:

- *Will chemo affect my fertility?*
- *Do I want biological children?*
- *Do I want the option, even if I'm not ready now?*

She was still single at the time.

So before chemo, she went through fertility preservation:

- Hormone injections
- Egg retrieval
- Freezing 16 eggs

Not romantic.

Not how anyone imagines planning for motherhood.

But deeply intentional. Another way of telling her future self, *"I've got you."*

Then came chemo.

Her regimen:

- Taxol
- Carboplatin

She did four rounds, with the week after each infusion being the hardest—physically and emotionally.

Instead of waiting for her hair to fall out in clumps in the shower, she chose to face it head-on.

She invited friends over.

They turned what could have been a traumatic moment into a communal, love-filled ritual.

Each friend cut a piece of her hair.

They laughed.

They took pictures.

They reframed loss as a shared act of care.

She shaved her head.

"I didn't want to be alone for that part. Making it a fun day helped me see it differently."

The People Who Stayed—and the Ones Who Fell Away

As her treatments unfolded, something else became clearer: who was truly in her corner.

Cancer has a way of shaking the tree of your life and letting the loose, dead fruit fall.

Chelsea began to see:

- Some friendships were solid, nourishing, and present.
- Others were based on convenience, social media performance, or drama.

Her mom was there.

Her twin sister was there—literally washing her, dressing her, helping her shower, holding drains, doing the intimate, unglamorous caregiving that strips away all pretense.

Her grandmother, at 93, had her own fears and old-school beliefs, worried how scars and reconstruction might affect Chelsea's chances of "finding a husband."

Chelsea listened.

Then she chose herself anyway.

She also noticed how people reacted online.

Sharing her journey on social media was a decision she wrestled with.

- Would it be "too much"?
- Would people judge?
- Would it make cancer feel more real?

She chose to share—openly and consistently—because awareness mattered to her.

What she got back was:

- Messages from people she hadn't spoken to since high school
- New friendships with women going through similar diagnoses across the country
- A sense of community she didn't know she needed

Her friends even organized a GoFundMe, and she watched, stunned and grateful, as donations trickled—and sometimes poured—in.

One of the most touching moments:

- Her oldest friend's father, whom she hadn't seen since childhood, donated $1,000 and sent an email so kind and heartfelt that she still cries when she re-reads it.

At the same time, she also saw who *didn't* show up.
Who had a lot of opinions but no real support.
Who used her story more as content than connection.
And quietly, she began to let those people go.

. . .

Love That Was There All Along: Jeff

If cancer exposed the weak links, it also illuminated something beautiful that had been right in front of her.

Jeff had been her friend for 10 years.

They'd joked since their early twenties that if they were both still single at 30, they'd get married. It was a half-serious, half-silly pact that lived in the background.

During her surgeries and chemo, Jeff didn't just send a "let me know if you need anything" text.

He showed up.

- He brought meals to her family after chemo.
- He checked in regularly.
- He came to visit her at her mom's house after her double mastectomy.

No grand gestures. Just quiet, steady presence.

Somewhere in the middle of the chaos, something clicked for Chelsea.

Before her last chemo, she took him out to dinner—not as a date, but as a thank-you.

Except it *became* a date.

She told him how she felt.

He told her he'd had a crush on her for nine years.

From there, their relationship grew into something solid and mutual.

Now they live together.

Jeff was one of the first people to see her bald, see her scarred, see her vulnerable.

Instead of pulling away, he leaned in.

That kind of love doesn't erase cancer.

It doesn't make chemo "worth it."

But it does become part of the story of how she emerged more deeply loved than before.

The Hardest Part Didn't Come During Chemo

For many people looking in from the outside, "the hard part" of cancer is obvious:

- Surgery
- Chemo
- Hair loss
- Nausea
- Scans

But for Chelsea, one of the hardest stretches came *after* treatment.

Once:

- The chemo ended,
- The surgeries were done,
- The drains were gone,
- Her hair started growing back...

Everybody else seemed to exhale and move on.

Chelsea expected to, too.

She thought, *"I'll just go back to work full-time and life will go back to normal."*

Instead, she found:

- Crying spells she couldn't explain

- Anxiety that spiked unexpectedly
- Insomnia and intense night sweats that soaked the sheets
- A body she barely recognized, after weight changes, meds, and hormonal shifts

She returned to work in a different department—a cold, competitive, negative environment where:

- People complained constantly,
- Some resented the accommodations she was given
- Coworkers whispered about her "special treatment"
  - Coming in late
  - Leaving early
  - Working from home when she didn't feel well

They saw:

- A full face of makeup
- A wig that looked like her old hair

They didn't see:

- The anxiety attacks
- The exhaustion
- The emotional whiplash of survivorship

Her bosses were supportive. They understood. But the overall energy of that department was toxic.
She tried therapy.
She tried different antidepressants.
She waited for things to "feel normal" again.
They didn't.
Because she wasn't the same person anymore.

Choosing Happiness Over "Progress"

Eventually, an opportunity surfaced:

Her old job—as office manager in the preschool—opened up again.

On paper, it looked like a step backward:

- Less "status"
- More support role, less management title

But in her body and her heart, it felt like absolute relief.

The preschool:

- Was warm and community-driven
- Felt like family
- Was filled with little humans who were unfiltered, loving, and unintimidated by her short curls

Her director wanted her back.

The school matched her salary.

The real question became:

"Do I want a fancier job title or a life I actually enjoy waking up for?"

Chelsea chose joy.

"People kept asking me, 'What's your goal from here?' And I said, 'To be happy.' I just went through cancer. I don't need a five-year career ladder plan right now. I need to love my life."

Back at the preschool, she:

- Felt alive again

- Laughed more
- Built healthier daily rhythms
- Let herself simply *be*

The kids didn't care about titles or corporate politics.

They cared about whether she would sit on the floor, color, listen, play, and show up as herself.

Her short curly hair became a source of connection—especially for little girls who'd never seen an adult woman with hair like theirs.

"When I straighten it, they tell me they like it better curly. They want me to look like them."

In that environment, her healing sped up.

What Cancer Changed—and What It Clarified

Chelsea will tell you she doesn't romanticize cancer.

She doesn't call it a blessing.

She doesn't pretend it wasn't terrifying, exhausting, and disruptive.

But she will say this:

It changed her:

- She no longer overbooks herself until she's running on fumes.
- She has learned to say no without drowning in guilt.
- She's become fiercely protective of her energy.
- She left friendships that were draining or performative.
- She doesn't chase people's approval the way she used to.

And it clarified what matters:

- Her health
- Her peace
- Her family
- Her relationship with Jeff
- A work environment that feels humane and joyful

She still lives with ongoing realities:

- Regular follow-ups
- BRCA-related ovarian risk and monitoring
- Night sweats and sleep challenges
- Emotional aftershocks that show up unexpectedly

But she carries them with a different posture now.
Not as a victim.
Not as someone who "failed" at prevention.
As a woman who listened to her intuition, caught an aggressive tumor early, and continues to choose herself—again and again.

Closing Reflection

Chelsea's journey asks an uncomfortable but liberating question:
What if the bravest thing you can do is stop living for everyone else's expectations and start living for your own well-being?
She refused to let other people's fears dictate her medical choices, refused to stay small to keep the peace, and refused to stay in a job that slowly eroded her spirit after she'd already fought so hard for her life.
Instead, she chose a different kind of "treatment plan":

- Radical self-care

- Honest boundaries
- Surrounding herself with people who show up
- Giving herself permission to be happy—even if it doesn't look impressive on a résumé

If you're standing at a crossroads—considering genetic testing, preventative surgery, a new doctor, a different job, or simply saying "no" more often—take a page from Chelsea. Trust the part of you that already knows what feels right, even if others don't understand.

Remember that healing doesn't end when chemo does; sometimes the hardest work begins after the last infusion, when the world expects you to "bounce back" and you're still figuring out who you are now.

You are allowed to choose peace over pressure, support over performance, and joy over just "getting through."

And like Chelsea, you are allowed to build a life that feels good from the inside out, even if it means rewriting every expectation you once held for yourself. Nearly six years have passed since our first interview, and in that time Chelsea and Jeff have married and welcomed a beautiful baby boy, Maddox—conceived through IVF using her frozen pre-chemo eggs. And now, in a twist that feels both miraculous and deeply earned, she is pregnant again, expecting another baby boy—this time conceived naturally.

Her story reminds us that hope does not vanish in the face of uncertainty; it simply waits for the moment when we are ready to believe in it again.

Chelsea's Grace Notes

- **Listening to your gut.**
    - Choosing a preventative double mastectomy at 30, despite others calling it "too drastic."

- Staying with an oncologist she trusted, instead of doctor-hopping every time someone else offered an opinion.
- **Reframing difficult moments as rituals.**
    - Turning head-shaving into a **gathering with friends**, making it about community instead of loss.
- **Intentional self-care (not the hashtag kind).**
    - Daily **bubble baths.**
    - Face masks.
    - Quiet time at home when she doesn't want to go out —without apologizing for it.
- **Choosing environment carefully.**
    - Leaving a toxic department even though it looked like a "step back" on paper.
    - Returning to the preschool where laughter, connection, and warmth became medicine.
- **Allowing help & practical support.**
    - Letting her twin sister shower and dress her.
    - Accepting meals, help, and financial support from friends, family, and strangers.
- **Sharing her story publicly.**
    - Posting about her journey on social media to build awareness and community.
    - Allowing herself to receive love, messages, and support from people far beyond her immediate circle.

The Art of Ordinary Miracles
Nicole's Story

How faith, family, and a two-year-old's dance party turned treatment into a different kind of grace.

Some stories arrive like lightning, others like a slow sunrise.

Nicole's began with an ordinary shower on an ordinary September day — soap, steam, a hand moving along a familiar path — and then a lump that shouldn't be there. A tiny interruption in the landscape of her body that would, in a matter of weeks, redraw almost everything.

What stayed, though, was the way she chose to see.

She didn't call it *luck*, and she didn't call it *battle*. Nicole reached for a different language — one of faith, of tiny provisions, of "coincidences" that didn't feel coincidental at all. Parents who had moved into her house just a month before diagnosis. A husband who landed a new job with a boss whose wife had just survived cancer. A church that wrapped her in prayer. A toddler who thought her bald head was just another thing to love.

In art, sometimes the most powerful pieces are built from very small marks, layered over time. Nicole's journey feels like that — an accumulation of ordinary miracles that, together, form a life that looks nothing like what she imagined and yet somehow feels fiercely, beautifully hers.

When Ordinary Cracked Open

In September 2019, 28-year-old Nicole found a lump in her right breast while showering. No drama, no ominous music — just a hand, a pause, a knowing that this didn't feel right.

She went to her doctor the same week. That single appointment unfolded into a chain: ultrasound, mammogram, more imaging, and eventually a series of biopsies — six in total, across both breasts.

By early October, she had a name for it: clinical stage I invasive ductal carcinoma in her right breast. The left side appeared benign.

In Dayton, the initial plan was swift and blunt: a double mastectomy, followed by dye testing during surgery to see whether cancer had reached her lymph nodes. No oncologist consult first. No multidisciplinary conversation. Just a surgery date.

Nicole liked the breast surgeon, but something in her resisted the pace.

"I wanted someone to step back and look at the whole picture," she explains.

So she did something critical: she slowed the story down.

She called The James at Ohio State University (OSU) for a second opinion. Within a week, she was in Columbus, and in a single day she met with a surgical oncologist, radiation oncologist, and medical oncologist — a full team.

The OSU surgeon looked at her Dayton records and shook his head gently.

"I don't even have enough information to put you on a surgery schedule," he told her. "We need more testing."

An MRI and additional imaging followed. This time, the scans told a different, harder truth:

Cancer had already reached her lymph nodes. A biopsy confirmed it. Her staging jumped from clinical Stage I to Stage III.

The plan changed with it. Surgery would wait. First, chemo.

Chemo First, and the Vanishing Spot

On November 12, 2019, Nicole sat down for her first infusion. The regimen was aggressive and intentional:

- 4 rounds of dose-dense AC (Adriamycin + Cytoxan)
- Followed by 4 rounds of dose-dense Taxol
- Treatments every two weeks

It was the "heavy hitter" protocol designed to shrink the tumor burden before anyone picked up a scalpel.

The chemo did what it was asked to do. Clinically, by the end of treatment:

- No one could feel the original lumps.
- A visible spot on her nipple — one of the first things that had screamed *this is wrong* to Nicole — had disappeared.

Her medical oncologist called it a "very good response." The final word will come only when the pathology report is back after surgery, but for now, the evidence is on her side.

Surgery is scheduled for March 16:

- Bilateral mastectomy
- Full lymph node dissection on the right (levels I & II)
- And, in a bold, proactive move: a prophylactic lymphovenous bypass performed by a plastic surgeon during the same operation.

Without that bypass, her risk of lymphedema — given her staging and full dissection — was estimated around 40%. The bypass, which reconnects severed lymphatic vessels directly into a nearby vein so fluid can drain into the venous system, could lower that risk to around 4%.

Some plastic surgeons only offer it after lymphedema appears. Nicole insisted on asking whether she could get ahead of it. One surgeon said no. Another said yes.

"I'm only 29," she told them. "I'm willing to try anything that gives me a better chance at a full life — without a compression sleeve for the next fifty years."

Insurance is still debating whether they'll cover this "newer" procedure. Nicole made peace with her own decision first:

She'll do it anyway. She'll figure out the rest.

A House, Already Full

A month before Nicole ever felt the lump, her parents sold their house.

Not on the market. Not after months of showings. They mentioned to a realtor that they *might* list, and a buyer appeared almost immediately. Suddenly they had nowhere to go while they planned their next move and future build. So, temporarily, they moved in with Nicole and her husband.

Thirty days later, she found the lump.

By the time chemo started, that "temporary" situation had quietly turned into one of the greatest gifts of her diagnosis.

Her mom became the heartbeat of the home — cooking, cleaning, watching their daughter Grace, folding herself into every gap that cancer tore open. When Nicole needed to rest, her mother handled everything. When Nicole felt well enough to load the dishwasher or sweep, her mom stepped back to give her that sense of normalcy and ownership.

"Sometimes you just need to wash your own dishes," Nicole says. "You need to remember this is still your life."

Her dad processed things differently. Talking about cancer didn't come easily, so his love came out as projects.

He finished their basement. He tackled home repairs. He built spaces Grace could play in and Nicole could recover in, as if to quietly say, *I can't fix this, but I can fix this.*

Her grandmother, just a minute away, watched Grace on infusion days, when Nicole, her mom, and her husband all drove to Columbus together.

Across the street, Nicole's sister — mom to three little girls — became the "second mother" in their growing village. Groceries showed up. Snacks appeared. Nieces shuffled in and out, filling the house with kid-noise that reminded everyone what they were fighting for.

And then there was work.

Nicole is a speech-language pathologist at a children's hospital, in a supervisor role that mixed patient care and administrative responsibilities. Her team and leadership didn't just offer sympathy; they redesigned her job around her treatment.

- No direct patient care during cold and flu season
- Hours cut from full-time to 20 hours per week
- Tasks reshaped into supervision, meetings, and projects she could do even when she was tired

Her hospital's employee assistance programs kicked in too: donated PTO, financial support, and a posture of *we've got you* that made it possible for her to keep receiving her regular paycheck without burning herself out.

Her rehab coworkers — speech, PT, OT — formed another layer of care. Every chemo day, a different group signed up to deliver a "chemo bag" of treats and comfort items. They organized meal trains so generous that Nicole eventually had to say, "You can slow down now. My freezer is full."

"I just keep seeing God's fingerprints on all of it," she says. "It's too many aligned details to be random."

Grace, Bald Heads, and Bedtime Kisses

When Nicole's oncologist talked about hair loss, he also talked about Grace.

Her daughter was 20 months old when all of this began — a toddler with opinions, routines, and a deep familiarity with Mom's long hair. He suggested they ease both of them into the change.

So two weeks before chemo started, Nicole cut her hair to chin-length. She came home braced for big feelings. Grace looked, blinked, touched the shorter ends, and went back to playing.

Fourteen days after the first infusion, the shedding began. Not catastrophic, but enough to make a mess and a point. On the day before Thanksgiving, she called her stylist.

"Let's buzz it," she said.

They shaved it down to a soft, even stubble — not quite bald, but close. She walked back into the house expecting at least a moment of confusion.

Grace toddled over, rubbed her mother's head like a new texture in a sensory bin, and grinned. Within days, kissing Mom's "soft head" became part of the bedtime ritual.

Kiss Mommy's head.
Mommy kisses Grace's head.
Grace kisses Daddy's head.
A tiny choreography of belonging, no matter what changed.

The port in Nicole's chest was harder for Grace to ignore. At first, everyone called it a "boo-boo," a visible reminder to be gentle when she climbed on Mom. As it healed, the warnings faded, but the word stuck — a toddler language that made medical hardware a little less scary.

Chemo shifted the family's emotional geography too.

Grace drifted into a Daddy's-girl season when bedtime stories, nighttime wake-ups, and big scoops into strong arms fell more often to him. Nicole watched it with something like relief and something like ache — but also with gratitude.

"It's a chance for their bond to deepen," she reminds herself. "And she'll find her way back to me again."

In the meantime, they dance.

Music on the Alexa. Living-room circles, little hands in big ones. Those few minutes of spinning and laughing and catching their breath are more than distraction — they are proof that joy is still here, threaded through the ordinary.

Faith, Anxiety, and the Shift From "Why Me?" to "What Now?"

When Nicole describes the months between finding the lump and getting a treatment plan, she doesn't sugarcoat it.

"I was anxious," she says simply. "I'm not usually an anxious person, but I was Googling everything, going down rabbit holes, imagining worst-case scenarios. I felt completely out of control."

What steadied her wasn't a guarantee of cure; it was a different kind of certainty.

She and her family are deeply rooted in their church. They serve, they show up, they sing. But cancer changed the texture of that faith from background to lifeline.

- Her pastor connected her immediately with a woman on the care ministry team who became a praying anchor — calling on the way to chemo, meeting for coffee, speaking calm over the chaos.
- She started staying after services to ask for private prayer, letting people anoint her and stand with her instead of slipping out quietly.
- She became intentional about reading Scripture, praying specifically, and letting others pray for her in detail too.

"I used to feel guilty asking for prayer," she admits. "I'd think, 'Other people have it worse.' Now I understand there's room for all of us."

Her understanding of "okay" changed too.

"Being okay doesn't mean I'm guaranteed a cure," she says. "It means I'm held, no matter what happens. That God is with me in it, whether healing comes here or on the other side of this life."

That belief doesn't erase scanxiety or bad days. But it gives her a way to talk back to fear.

When she catches herself spiraling about recurrence — every twinge, every cough, every ache — she comes back to a simple, fierce truth:

- *My team is doing everything they can.*
- *I'm doing everything I can.*

- *If the cancer comes back, it will not be because I failed.*

Worrying about tomorrow doesn't buy her more time. It only steals today.

So she practices small acts of trust — planning Disney now instead of "in a few years," enrolling Grace in swim lessons and gymnastics during chemo instead of waiting for some mythical "better time," and choosing to see each weekday not as something to get through but as something she *gets* to live.

"Thursday is just as precious as Saturday now," she says. "I don't live for the weekend anymore."

Learning to Ask, Learning to Receive

Nicole laughs when she talks about how stubborn she used to be about help.

"I'm the helper," she says. "I don't like being the one who needs."

Cancer dismantled that identity in ways both humbling and holy.

- She told her leadership at work she needed reduced hours and no patient care — and they said yes.
- She let coworkers organize meals, chemo bags, and future rides to radiation.
- She opened the door when organizations like Pink Ribbon Girls stepped in with chef-prepared frozen meals and professional house cleaning, even when part of her brain said, *You could still cook...*

Online, she navigated support groups carefully, learning how to hold other people's pain without drowning in it. "Cancer is a Mother," HER2+ communities, and "flat & fabulous" groups offered practical tips, fashion ideas for living flat, and occasional heartbreak.

She learned to visit with intention:

- Go in with a question or purpose.
- Take what's helpful.
- Step back when it becomes too heavy.

And she did something else that scared her more than any Facebook post: she let people pray *specifically* for her.

"I even give them details now," she says. "'Please pray that my nodes are clear. Please pray for my surgery date.'"

Asking didn't make her weak. It made her honest. And in that honesty, she found community she hadn't realized was waiting for her.

Closing Reflection

Nicole's story is not tidy. There are still scans ahead, surgeries to heal from, radiation to endure, and the long unknown of survivorship stretching out like an unfinished canvas.

But when I think of her, what rises first is not the pathology or the protocols. It's the picture of a young woman with a shaved head and a toddler on her hip, spinning under soft living-room light, laughing, breathless, fully present.

A mother letting herself be loved by parents who moved in "just for a while," by coworkers who fill her freezer, by a husband who will talk about Girl Scouts and future birthdays even when it hurts his heart.

A woman of faith who no longer confuses "being okay" with "being guaranteed a miracle" — and yet still chooses to see miracles in a finished basement, a lymph node-saving surgery, a church prayer chain, a day at work, a kiss on a bald head.

If art is, at its core, the act of paying attention and turning what we notice into meaning, then Nicole is living art. Her life right now is a collage of scans and Sharpied radiation fields, snack cups and dance parties, IV pumps and bedtime kisses.

And in the middle of all of it, she keeps practicing her craft: Waking up each morning and saying, *I get to be here.*

Trusting that even in chemo chairs and pre-op rooms, ordinary miracles are still being stitched into her days.

Nicole's Grace Notes

- **Get the whole orchestra, not just one instrument.** If something in your plan doesn't sit right, listen to that nudge. Nicole's second opinion at OSU completely changed her staging and treatment. Seek a multidisciplinary team — surgical, medical, and radiation oncology together — before major decisions.
- **Ask about proactive options, even if they sound "too advanced."** Her prophylactic lymphovenous bypass wasn't offered at first; she had to ask and then ask again. Whether it's surgical techniques, clinical trials, or side-effect management, it's okay to say, *"Is there anything else we can do?"*
- **Build your village early and let it help.** Family, coworkers, church, neighbors, organizations like Pink Ribbon Girls — they want to show up. Let them. Meals, rides, cleaning, childcare — every task someone else carries gives your body more room to heal.
- **Protect your mind as much as your body.** Online groups can be lifelines *and* landmines. Use them

strategically: look for resources, local connections, and practical hacks, and step away when posts pull you into fear instead of strength.

- **Keep living *during* treatment, not just after.** Chemo didn't make Nicole hit "pause" on life. She worked part-time, planned trips, signed Grace up for activities, and kept as many daily rhythms as her energy allowed. You're not just a patient; you're still a person.
- **Name what cancer has given you, not just what it has taken.** For Nicole, that list includes:
  - A deeper relationship with God.
  - A sharper sense of time's preciousness.
  - The ability to ask for — and receive — help.
  - A new tenderness for other people's pain.
  - A thousand small moments with her daughter she might have otherwise rushed past.

The Art of Holding Two Lives
Maria's Story

Sometimes courage is painted in the space between fear and faith.

"I was carrying a baby and a diagnosis at the same time—
    so I chose to love both, one breath, one infusion, one ordinary day at a time."

A Knock That Changed Everything

Some phone calls divide life into *before* and *after*.

For Maria, it came at eleven weeks pregnant—with young children tugging at her sleeves and the smell of oatmeal still warm in the air. Her midwife wanted her to come in "to review results." When Maria asked if it could wait, the nurse hesitated: *"She really wants to see you."*

That pause said everything.

At the clinic, she balanced a diaper bag on her knee and tried to keep the boys entertained. The midwife closed the door, took a breath, and spoke: *"It's invasive ductal carcinoma."*

Maria blinked once. "You've got to be kidding me."

Then, quieter, almost to herself: *"I don't have time for this."*

Those five words—half fury, half defiance—became her first act of survival.

Two Heartbeats, One War

At twenty-seven, Maria was carrying her third child and the weight of an uninvited disease. Tests later confirmed the most aggressive subtype—*triple-negative breast cancer*. Because of the pregnancy, doctors couldn't perform full-body scans. "We'll call it Stage III," they said gently, "and confirm later."

The days blurred between oncology appointments and prenatal checkups. Her body became a meeting ground for two kinds of life: one growing, one trying to take root where it didn't belong.

When she checked into Moffitt Cancer Center in Tampa, she wasn't alone. She carried her unborn son's heartbeat inside her—proof that hope could share space with fear.

Surgeons performed a unilateral mastectomy. The anesthesia had to be carefully timed, the baby constantly monitored. They couldn't remove both breasts yet—it was too risky for her tiny passenger. The rest would have to wait.

Then came the "Red Devil," Adriamycin, and Cytoxan—chemo cocktails so toxic the nurses wore gloves to handle them. It was December. While most families hung ornaments and baked cookies, Maria was learning to steady her breathing between infusions.

She remembers thinking, *This isn't how pregnancy is supposed to feel.*

And yet, somewhere in the sterile rhythm of IV drips, life kept happening. Kicks beneath her ribs. Ultrasound prints on the fridge. Two toddlers giggling in the next room. The world did not pause, and so neither did she.

The Warrior Beside Her

Maria's husband, a combat veteran, had already faced fear in other landscapes. This time, the battlefield was home.

He never asked how she felt—he simply acted. "Up. Shower. Shoes."

On chemo Fridays, they'd walk the aisles of Target, or stroll Disney as annual pass holders, pretending for an hour that they were just another family in the sunshine.

"I wasn't allowed to fall apart," Maria says. "He wouldn't let me."

That's love in its truest form—not the cinematic kind, but the quiet insistence of partnership. The one who hands you your strength when you can't find it.

When her hair began to fall, he brought the clippers. The boys watched from the couch, their eyes wide but unafraid. To them, it wasn't tragedy—it was family haircut day. Maria smiled for them. She'd shaved half her head once before for a mohawk; this time, she went all in.

Losing the eyebrows and lashes hit harder. "That's when I *looked* like a cancer patient," she says softly. "And that word... even now... it hurts to say."

Still, she painted on eyeliner, swiped lipstick across pale lips, and showed up. Motherhood doesn't allow many sick days. "I didn't want my boys to remember me in bed. I wanted them to remember I kept moving."

Community in the Dark Hours

Her oncologist had treated other pregnant patients before her and connected them. That introduction led her to a private Facebook group—Kick Ass Cancer Mamas—where a hundred women across continents shared both science and solace.

It became her lifeline at 2 a.m. when nausea, fear, and fetal kicks collided. There, she could say the unsayable—to women who understood what it meant to feel both blessed and betrayed by your own body.

Through them she learned the strange solidarity of this sisterhood: how you could mourn and laugh in the same breath; how hope multiplied when spoken aloud.

Among them was *Karina*, whose baby girl was born just weeks apart from Maria's son. They met once in person at a Panera Bread near the oncology office—two mothers comparing chemo notes over soup. Months later, Karina's cancer metastasized. Then she was gone.

"It was a punch in the gut," Maria says. "Because she was right there. Because she was me."

That loss could have broken her. Instead, it became a vow: to live wide open. To honor the fallen by refusing to vanish into grief.

Choosing Presence Over Perfection

Before cancer, Maria lived by lists. Type-A efficiency. A clean sink meant peace; clutter meant chaos. After cancer, the definition of "done" changed.

"The dishes don't matter anymore," she says. "The counter can stay messy. I'd rather watch a movie in our pajamas or sneak away to Disney midweek. That's what time well spent looks like now."

She stopped confusing busyness with purpose. She started measuring her days in laughter and rest, not productivity.

And yet, this wasn't complacency—it was clarity. "I used to think doing more meant living more," she says. "Now I know the most important things don't show up on a checklist."

Fear, Revisited

Even with NED stamped on her chart—*no evidence of disease*—the echoes remain.

Recently, after a minor car accident, an X-ray showed dark spots. Her stomach dropped. *It's back,* she thought. Panic climbed like static until she sent the images to a nurse friend. The reply came minutes later: *"Sweetheart, those are gas bubbles."*

Maria laughed through tears. Fear had borrowed the mic again, but she knew how to turn the volume down.

"When I get scared now, I let myself feel it," she says. "Then I say, 'Okay, you can sit here, but you can't stay.' I don't shove it away—but I don't feed it either."

She learned that naming fear gives it shape, and once something has shape, it can be faced.

The Paperwork of Love

. . .

Years before cancer, a recurring nightmare about dying during childbirth pushed Maria to write a will and get life insurance. When cancer came, she simply updated the binder. Guardianship plans. Mortgage payoff instructions. Funds for a nanny so her husband could keep working.

"I took control of what I could," she says. "Then I closed the drawer."

That small act—*organize, then release*—became her philosophy. Preparation gave her permission to live.

The Miracle of Two Lives

When her son was born at 39 weeks, the delivery room was crowded with both OBs and oncology specialists. The moment he cried, Maria exhaled a prayer she didn't know she'd been holding.

Tests later revealed no cancer cells in her placenta. Her oncologist explained that certain chemo molecules are too large to cross the barrier—"your placenta built a gate," he said.

Maria still calls it a miracle. "My body fought for both of us," she says. "It built a wall to keep him safe."

Today, that boy is eight—healthy, fearless, and full of laughter. Maria watches him mature and thinks, *You were the reason I never stopped.*

Closing Reflection

Cancer didn't make Maria grateful overnight. It stripped her bare first. Gratitude came slowly, like sunlight returning after a storm—subtle, but steady.

She learned that gratitude isn't about pretending pain doesn't exist. It's about widening your gaze enough to see both—the loss *and* the light.

So she paints her days differently now: slower strokes, more pauses, richer color. A little lipstick on a chemo face. A messy counter beside a giggling child. A walk through Disney with tired feet but a full heart.

That's the art of survival—and of living.

Maria's Grace Notes

- **Move before the crash.** On infusion weekends, plan gentle outings before side effects peak. Motion keeps your spirit awake.
- **Find your people.** Prioritize your oncology nurse and social worker for real help; lean on groups like *Kick Ass Cancer Mamas*—especially across time zones for the 3 a.m. spirals.
- **Prepare, then release.** Handle wills, insurance, and care plans early, then set them aside. Life deserves your presence, not your panic.
- **Speak your fear aloud.** Silence grows monsters. Saying it shrinks them.
- **Redefine productivity.** Clean kitchens fade; memories don't. Choose presence over perfection.

The Art of Permission
Sara's Story

When *urgency becomes permission — and permission becomes a life worth living.*

It was a quiet Sunday morning, the kind where steam curls from a coffee mug and the house hasn't quite woken up. We sat together on video—me with my notebook, Sara with her cup—and named the thing we both know: young mothers with cancer are too often left out of the frame. The literature, the support rooms, the tone of it all—they skew older. But here we were, the same age, the same ache for a life that's big and bright for our kids and ourselves. She said "thrive," and I felt the word land like a key turning in a lock.

In September 2012, at thirty-four, Sara was diagnosed with stage IIIA invasive ductal carcinoma. Five tumors in her right breast, the largest three-and-a-half centimeters. Within five days of hearing the word "cancer," she was on the table for an emergency mastectomy. Then came eight rounds of chemotherapy, thirty-six radiation treatments, four surgeries. Tamoxifen for a decade; Lupron for two grueling years until quality of life finally said "enough." Today, seven-plus years out from diagnosis, she's here—still a wife, still a mother, still a teacher—and something else too: more herself than she's ever been.

The Moment Everything Shifted

She had just come through back-to-back babies—twenty months and three years—and could map the midwife's office by heart. Healthy. Active. Yoga, running, non-smoker. "I didn't fit the picture," she said, and yet the picture changed anyway. By the time imaging laid the truth bare, her right breast was crowded with five distinct masses. "If it's that big," she remembers thinking, "how hasn't it spread everywhere?" Fear rushed in, swift and certain. And still, the body did what bodies do: it healed, one decision, one infusion, one recovery day at a time.

Motherhood, mid-treatment

There is nothing theoretical about mothering small children while your chest is bandaged and your scalp goes smooth. You still remind them to be gentle. You still manage snacks, naps, drop-offs. And when they ask why Mommy has a scar, you answer simply, truth scaled to their age: "Mommy had surgery." Because sometimes the kindest way through is the plainest.

Years later—now nine and ten—her boys know the fuller story. They vaguely remember the baldness; what they carry most, though, is the climate of their home: openness without dread, honesty without spectacle. When one asked, softly, "Can cancer come back?"

she told the truth the way a mother does: with care and a steady gaze. "Anyone can get sick, but I'm okay right now." Sometimes the best gift we give our children is a nervous system that refuses to catastrophize.

The Internal Rearranging

"I thought I was wimpy," Sara laughed, surprised at her own sentence. Cancer reordered that story. Pain pills largely went unused. Anxiety, yes. But under it, a deeper current: strength. "Nothing hurt as badly as I thought it would." Strength became confidence; confidence turned into permission. Permission to live more authentically. Permission to stop pleasing on autopilot. Permission to become the author of her one life.

The chrysanthemum on her arm—her November birth flower—wasn't rebellion so much as a vow. At thirty-five, she did the thing she wanted because she wanted it. Not to perform grit, but to honor it.

Time: The Tender Paradox

"The problem is, you think you have time." The quote found her and wouldn't let go. Post-treatment, time split open: urgency married to gratitude. On one side—racing the clock, the mind's fast math of recurrence risk. On the other—the holy ordinary of a life she refuses to spend in fear. She names both. She chooses presence anyway. Walks with the dogs. Eyeliner on days she feels gray. Dancing with her boys in the kitchen. A life worth living isn't an accident; it's a practice.

. . .

Relationships In A New Light

Cancer is a sieve. The unexpected ones show up (a high-school friend at the door with hot food, two decades later); the expected ones sometimes don't. Marriage goes through the ringer. Some friendships molt and don't grow back. Boundaries sharpen. Authenticity becomes a quiet, daily choreography: what serves, stays; what drains, goes. She has less appetite for performance—hers or anyone else's. There's a dog-whistle frequency to inauthenticity now; she hears it, and she steps away.

Making meaning (on purpose)

She began a blog to keep people updated, and it quickly turned into truth-telling. Not a glossy arc—just the interior weather of a body and mind in repair. Writing pulled her back to herself. Painting, too— "I'm not 'good,' but I love it," she says, which is exactly the point. Yoga, breathwork, walking, gentler self-talk in the mirror. None of it is a cure. All of it is medicine.

"*I didn't go through all of that to be miserable,*" she told me, and something in me stood up straighter. We get to curate the inputs. We get to choose the rituals. We get to claim a nervous system that believes in morning.

Finding Rooms That Fit

Most pamphlets felt like they were written for someone else's mother. So she kept looking. The Young Survival Coalition's annual conference (for women diagnosed under 40) became a lifeline: speakers, movement, a Saturday night dance floor where joy wasn't a betrayal of grief. She saw women at every stage—diagnosis to thriving—and something unclenched. There is a future. There are rooms like this.

She points others to Living Beyond Breast Cancer for practical content, to Stupid Cancer for young-adult cancer community, and to secular spaces where care doesn't arrive wrapped in platitudes she doesn't share. Peer support matters; so, does fit. Sometimes the most spiritual thing you can do is find a room that lets you exhale.

What Cancer Gave (and what it didn't)

She resists the easy "gift" language, but she also won't deny what's true: a sturdier self-love; a clearer sense of what matters (experiences over stuff, memories over more); permission to be fully Sara. The external trappings of her life returned—classroom keys jangling again, lunchboxes packed. The inside is where the renovation holds.

And the fear? It visits. A recent car accident, an X-ray shadow that sent her spiraling until a nurse friend texted back, "Those are gas bubbles, love." She laughed, then breathed, then kept going. Naming fear is part of honoring life. Letting it steer is not.

Closing Reflection

Not every story needs a battle cry. Some ask for a softer bravery—the kind that gets the kids to school, answers the hard questions gently, paints anyway, and chooses joy without betraying the truth. Listening to Sara, I kept thinking: this is what healing can look like when urgency becomes permission. Not louder—truer. Not faster—

fuller. A life measured less by what was taken and more by what was finally allowed.

Sara's Grace Notes

- **Let urgency become permission.** Stop waiting for a better time to be yourself. Do the thing. Book the trip. Dance on the Saturday night of a cancer conference.
- **Curate your inputs.** Gentle self-talk. Yoga, walks, paint on your hands, words on a page. None of it is performative; all of it is nervous-system care.
- **Find the right room.** Seek peers your age/stage. Try **Young Survival Coalition**, **Living Beyond Breast Cancer**, and **Stupid Cancer**. Keep what serves; drop what doesn't.
- **Speak simply to your kids.** Age-appropriate, calm, honest. "Mommy had surgery." As they grow, let their questions lead.
- **Rebuild your circle.** Notice who shows up. Set boundaries without apology. Authenticity is an act of health.
- **Work with time, not against it.** Name the paradox —gratitude and urgency—and then choose presence on purpose.
- **Use your care team strategically.** Oncologist for plans; nurse and oncology social worker for speed and support. Skip Dr. Google.
- **Quality of life counts.** If a medication drains you beyond reason, ask about alternatives. Feeling alive is part of staying alive.

The Art of Living Out Loud
Stephanie's Story

E*ven when tomorrow feels uncertain, today is still a masterpiece.*

Every canvas holds a moment when the artist must choose: pause in fear of the next brushstroke, or lay down color anyway. Stephanie's story is that brave, decisive stroke—laid on thick, unapologetic, and full of life. In her, I see the practice of gratitude not as a quiet whisper, but as a bright pigment cut through with humor and grit. She paints with what she has: a five-year-old boy's questions, a coastline's wind, music turned up too loud, and a heart that refuses to stop making memories. This is the art of living out loud—of choosing vibrancy in the face of uncertainty, and love in the face of loss.

Declaring your truth, the good, bad, and ugly

. . .

When Stephanie felt the lump, she was twenty-nine and already fluent in the language of split-second adjustment: a toddler on her hip, co-parenting with her ex-husband, a full-time job in the animal world, and a relationship that would soon show its darker edges. The date fixed itself in memory—March 28, 2017—the day the horizon line shifted. Doctors called it stage 2B breast cancer. Tumors clustered in her left breast; disease hid in a lymph node beneath her arm. Even then, Stephanie sensed more was moving under the surface than the scans could catch.

She did what mothers do. She acted.

Aggressive treatment. A double mastectomy—her choice, despite mixed messages from clinicians who weighed youth against risk. Ports, drains, pain. Chemo that rearranges the calendar and the mirror. And then the revelation that ends more than one kind of suffering: while the surgical drains still clung to her skin, the man she was with put hands on her. She left—walked out, bandaged and unbowed, and went to her brother's. Courage, sometimes, is as practical as a packed bag and a front door closing.

For a brief stretch, hope settled in. A staff member in her doctor's office called with the words every patient learns to pronounce like a fragile spell: "no evidence of disease." Stephanie's little boy was nearby—eyes shining—and she let herself celebrate out loud. They hugged, they laughed, they took up space in happiness because joy, like grief, needs a body to live in.

Months later, on the cusp of her one-year cancerversary, the room went still.

A nurse practitioner sat down and said it like a weather report: "We're restaging you to stage 4 metastatic breast cancer."

No soft landing. No measured preface. Just the new fact of it: the cancer had traveled beyond the breast and nodes. It would require a different kind of living.

Stephanie didn't cry then. She watched her mother and grandmother cry. She listened for the next instruction. She took treatment that day.

Telling her son—Knox, four at the time—required a different vocabulary. When he was two, the explanations were simple: *Mama is sick. The medicine makes my hair fall out.* He learned to hold clumps of hair without fear. When he was older, she gave him a metaphor a child could carry: *"Chemotherapy is a bunch of tiny guns that shoot the bad stuff."* It made sense to him. It made sense to her. Kids see through the fog when we give them a lantern.

Stephanie refused to disappear from his daily life. Doctors warned her about germs and school drop-offs; she nodded and showed up anyway. *I was made to be a mom,* she says. *Now I'm a mom fighting an incurable disease.* The sentence is both burden and banner, and she holds it like a standard in a parade of ordinary days: breakfast, backpacks, car lines, bedtime. Presence, more than perfection, is the point.

In the quiet moments, the story expands.

There's Corpus Christi wind in her hair and ocean salt drying on her skin. She has surfed since she was two; now she imagines teaching Knox to read the water the way she does—by feel, by faith. There are dance parties in the living room and reggae turned up until the walls remember joy. Sublime, Beastie Boys, today's hits—whatever loosens grief's grip for a few minutes. Music, like medicine, changes the chemistry of a room.

There are scars that itch and ache where the cancer has done what no one warned her it might do: metastasize to the skin. Heat, redness, the shock of seeing new lumps bloom after a biopsy, the texture turning hard where surgeons borrowed tissue from her back to build a new shape of her chest. She has known the antiseptic loneliness of a month in the hospital fighting an infection with "heavy-duty" antibiotics, the way plastic expands and skin contracts, the way anger can flare and settle like a storm.

Now comes a next line on the treatment map: Kadcyla (she grins at how she says it, then shrugs—*cad-sila, close enough*). It promises, not certainty, but possibility. She reads every side effect. She hopes anyway. That is the hard choreography of stage 4: learn the steps, improvise, keep moving.

Cancer rearranged her relationships as surely as it rearranged her cells.

Some ties tightened: her ex-husband James and she now co-parent under one roof, building a stable, loving orbit for Knox. Other ties broke: painful words from her mother and grandmother drew a boundary she refuses to cross. Protecting her son from harm—present or potential—isn't cruelty; it's clarity.

The diagnosis didn't make Stephanie a different person; it made her a truer one. When a second opinion estimated "two to three years," she didn't collapse. She decided. She shifted her life from later to now.

It shows up in little things that are not little: the pre lit fake Christmas tree she chose because one day, if she isn't there, father and son can unbox it and say *we picked this with Mom*. It shows up in the gloves she took off at a drive-thru to warm the cashier's hands, in the $100 bill she slipped to a courteous store employee just because good manners felt like a light the world should reward. It shows up in how she shops for Knox's room—curtains, a sturdy bed, small pieces of permanence—so he'll be surrounded by *Mom's choices* as much as her memories.

It shows up in the keepsakes she is quietly crafting: messages and notes, a journal she opens when courage arrives, a Kept/"Keepsake" app that pings twice a day—*What would you like to tell your son today?*—and compiles the answers into a book. She buys cards for future milestones because presence can be prewritten. She records videos when she can bear seeing her own face. These are not morbid acts; they are loving ones. They are brushstrokes on a canvas meant to last.

She laughs easily, sometimes darkly, because humor is oxygen in tight spaces.

"Keep your humor," she tells other parents. "If I walk around saying I'm dying in three years, then the room dies with me." So she refuses. She names the hard truth—and then cracks a joke to let the light back in.

There's a fierceness to her advocacy that's part lioness, part lawyer. She reads her own scans. She calls her doctor's office instead of waiting by the phone. She knows the meanings of *PET*, *Herceptin*, *Perjeta*, *echocardiogram*, and she knows when a sentence lands wrong and needs a follow-up question. She tells women who message her—*Go to your doctor. Don't WebMD this. Ask for answers. This is your body, not a suggestion box.* Self-advocacy, for Stephanie, is not about control as much as it is about dignity.

And yet presence, not planning, is what steadies her most. When anxiety spikes, she steps outside and looks up. Breath in. Sun on skin. *I'm alive right now.* The simple sentence is a prayer. Gratitude, in her hands, isn't a performance. It's a practice.

She won't pretend she doesn't grieve—especially in the shower, where the water hides tears. Some nights she crawls straight into bed and lets the noise of fear quiet itself by fading, not fighting. Strength and softness can live in the same body. So can anger and amazement. So can the ache of what's coming and the joy of a five-year-old's dance break at 7:13 p.m. on a Tuesday.

The art of living out loud is not the absence of pain; it's the refusal to mute the love that remains.

Closing Reflection

. . .

Stephanie reminds me that gratitude can be bright and bold—paint splashed across a wall where fear once hung like a curtain. Her courage isn't tidy; it's textured. It looks like surfboards waiting by a door, like a pre-lit tree ready to anchor a holiday, like a mother who will not apologize for loving loudly while she can.

As an artist, I know a finished piece is never free of mistakes—it's full of them, transformed. Stephanie does that with her days. She turns interruptions into invitations: to laugh, to give, to prepare, to be present, to dance. She makes a masterpiece out of the hours she has, then signs it with gratitude so her son will always know how it felt to be loved by her.

It is with great sorrow that Stephanie passed away from cancer prior to this book being published. May her memory be a blessing and her legacy live on through the stories her family shares.

Stephanie's Grace Notes

- **Keep your humor.** Laughter breaks the fear spiral and gives kids permission to be kids.
- **Explain honestly, simply, and often.** Age-appropriate language works: "the medicine shoots the bad stuff." Loop in teachers/counselors.
- **Be your own advocate.** Read reports, call for results, ask follow-ups, and push for clarity. This is your body and your life.
- **Choose presence over perfection.** Show up for drop-offs, dance parties, and small rituals. Your child needs you present, not flawless.
- **Make memories now.** Plan the girls' trip. Play the music loud. Eat the dessert. The calendar can be a work of art.

- **Prepare with love, not fear.** Write letters, record messages, label keepsakes, pre-plan logistics (wills, plots, finances) to lighten future burdens.
- **Protect your peace.** Set boundaries with anyone who brings harm or chaos. Curate a circle that adds love to your child's world.
- **Find a grounding ritual.** Step outside, look up, breathe. Name one thing you're grateful for—sun warmth, a silly song, a clean scan, a stale cracker that still helped.
- **Let help in.** Friends, co-parents, neighbors—allow them to carry pieces of the load so you can carry the parts only you can.
- **Trust your body wisdom.** Do self-exams, follow your instincts, and seek evaluation for new or lingering symptoms—early attention matters.

The Art of Holding On and Letting Go
Carrie's Story

Strength is not always loud. Sometimes it's the quiet choice to rise again.

Some lives look like a clean, elegant routine: you run, leap, land, and the crowd claps on cue.

Others look more like what happens after the music stops—when you're on the mat, wind knocked out of you, and the only art left is the art of getting back up.

Carrie's story is not a tidy, framed canvas. It's more like a series of chalk-dusted handprints along a balance beam: slips, wobbles, deep breaths, and that fierce decision—over and over—to stay on.

She learned early how to live with unanswered questions. Adopted as a baby into a loving family, she grew up already knowing that life can begin in uncertainty and still become beautiful. Maybe that's why, when cancer slammed into her at twenty-eight—just as she was stepping into her adult life, managing a preschool and coaching gymnastics—some deep part of her already knew how to adapt. To take what was given and still make something out of it.

Art and gratitude, for Carrie, aren't soft feelings. They're disciplines. They show up in the way she chooses routine over chaos, community over isolation, and a thousand small acts of care over one grand gesture. They show up in a shaved-head party in a gym full of little girls, in a banquet hall packed with people who adore her, in a coloring book she opens one page at a time with her five-year-old son.

Her life is the art of holding on and letting go at the same time—holding on to hope, to Nicholas, to ordinary days; letting go of certainty, timelines, and the illusion that control is the same thing as safety.

This is her story.

What Carrie Teaches Us About Fierce Tenderness

Carrie was twenty-eight and "twenty-eight years *young*," as she likes to say, when she first heard the words.

She had just graduated college. She was managing a preschool in a gymnastics studio, coaching kids on beams and bars, single, dating here and there, and doing that quiet, invisible work of growing up—stepping out of her twenties and toward her thirties.

It started on an ordinary Friday night in the shower.

Her hand slid under her right arm in that familiar, thoughtless movement we all make when we wash—and stopped.

There was a lump.

She didn't know much about breast cancer back then. Sixteen years ago, it didn't saturate the culture the way it does now. At twenty-eight, it certainly wasn't on her personal radar. Her first thought wasn't doom; it was more like *huh, that's weird*.

Over the weekend, she mentioned it to her mom, her partner in everything even then. "It's probably just a cyst," her mom said. "Hormonal." Still, on Monday, Carrie did the thing that would later feel like the first of many brave, ordinary acts: she followed up. She went to her primary care doctor.

From there, everything snowballed.

There was the ultrasound. Then the first time the word *cancer* floated into the room—not as a sentence, but as a possibility: *could be benign, could be malignant.* There was the biopsy. And then, one early morning at 8:30 a.m., the phone rang.

"Carrie, you have breast cancer."

She remembers the way her body reacted before her mind did—how she threw the phone, how her mom picked it up, how she retreated to her room and sat there, stunned. She knew chemo meant hair loss, fatigue, nausea. But the rest? The staging, the pathology, HER2, receptors, acronyms that sound like another language—none of that had a shape yet.

Within weeks, her world had been reorganized around appointments: oncologist, surgeon, second opinion. Massive choices came at her like a barrage—lumpectomy or mastectomy? Bilateral? Radiation? How aggressive do we go?

Her mother became her note-taker, her filter, her second brain. While Carrie was still trying to breathe, her mom listened, translated, and quietly helped her walk through the decisions.

Eventually, the picture sharpened:

Stage III invasive ductal carcinoma. HER2 positive. Aggressive.

The HER2 news landed like a punch. "We're hoping it's not HER2 positive," someone had said, "because that's a very aggressive subtype with a poorer prognosis." It was HER2 positive.

On the day she heard that, she lay back on the exam table, her mom and three aunts ringed around her like a wall of love. The oncologist, not warm in the Hallmark-movie sense, but solid, knowledgeable, and sure, took her hands.

"I think I'm going to die," she said out loud.

The oncologist looked her straight in the eyes.

"No, Carrie. You're not going to die. It just means we're going to treat this very aggressively."

So they did.

Six months of Adriamycin and Cytoxan—the red devil and its equally brutal partner. Taxol. Thirty-five rounds of radiation. A lumpectomy. Steroids. Endless waiting rooms and blood draws. Side effects piling on: exhaustion, nausea, and later, years of severe GI motility issues that would require stomach surgery and steal nearly five more years of feeling well.

Before she could grieve the possible loss of her fertility, the medical urgency answered that question for her. She was twenty-eight, single, aggressively HER2 positive, and needed chemo *now*. There wasn't time to harvest eggs. The conversation was brief, almost academic—here are some options, here's the reality—and then they were already wheeling her toward the treatment that might save her life.

Because she'd been adopted as an infant, she carried, deep in her bones, the living proof that biology isn't the only way to become a mother. "I knew," she says, "that if I survived, I could always give a child a home." She let that knowing steady her as she chose survival first.

Through it all, her village showed up.

Her best friend Patty, who owned the gymnastics gym and had been Carrie's coach since she was eight, refused to let cancer steal everything. "Come to work," she'd say. "Just come. Once you're here, you'll forget for a little while."

There were days when Carrie didn't want to move. But she would drag herself to the gym, and for those hours she wasn't "the girl with cancer." She was Coach Carrie, keeping kids safe on the beam, spotting handstands, barking corrections and cheering routines. The gym became, in its own way, a studio—one where the art was presence, and the medium was other people's joy.

When her long black hair began coming out in clumps, she didn't shave it alone in a bathroom. They threw a shaving party.

One night at the gym, friends gathered with razors and bandanas. Some of the kids placed pieces of duct tape on small patches of her hair and tugged them off, turning the horror of hair loss into something weirdly funny and communal. It wasn't the private, sobbing scene she'd dreaded. It was messy, loud, and loving.

The wigs—sitting in a salon full of older women, feeling like an imposter, trying on other people's hair—had made her cry. The shaving party made her feel held.

Radiation came next and left a different kind of mark. The burns on her skin were bad, but it was the exhaustion and throat pain that nearly broke her. The beams scorched the bottom of her esophagus; swallowing felt like fire. IV fluids, hospital stays, a body that seemed to be running on fumes. By the thirty-something session, her team told her, "You've done enough. You can stop."

The overachiever in her wanted to finish all thirty-five. But the woman who had learned, the hard way, that listening to her body was not weakness, allowed herself to stop. Even then, in that small act of mercy, there was art: the art of letting go of a rigid idea of "completion" in order to honor a living, breathing self.

Then came the long aftermath.

The cancer, eventually, went quiet. The scans cleared. But the motility problems roared. For almost four and a half years, she was medically fragile in a way no one puts on t-shirts. Her stomach didn't work properly. Eating, digesting, simply existing felt like another ordeal. She was sick of being sick.

Only around ten years out—after GI surgery, slow healing, and countless appointments—did she finally exhale. The panic that flared with every cold or random pain softened. She began to use the "two-week rule": wait, watch, then call, instead of sprinting to worst-case scenarios. For the first time since her twenties, she felt like herself again.

She went back to school. She started working as a nursing assistant at Boston Children's Hospital, on the pediatric trauma floor—a job that demanded thick skin, big heart, and a tolerance for chaos. She had all three. She excelled there. She thought cancer, while always part of her story, was now a closed chapter.

And then 2016 happened.

It began as something so ordinary it was almost laughable: laryngitis. She lost her voice in October and assumed what everyone around her did—it was viral, seasonal, a hazard of working in a hospital full of sick kids. She saw her doctor multiple times and heard the same thing: it's a cold, it's going around, you're fine.

But the laryngitis didn't leave. Eight, nine weeks went by.

At the end of October, she was working with an autistic teenager when he suddenly became aggressive and knocked an IV pole—loaded with pumps—onto her back, driving her to the floor and knocking the wind out of her. She was shaken, sore, and sent for an X-ray to check for injuries.

The X-ray caught something else.

A shadow, an oddity in her chest. Maybe a contusion from the impact; maybe not. "Follow up," they said.

By late November, still hoarse, now with chest pain and trouble swallowing, something inside her snapped into that old, familiar clarity. She drove herself into Boston and insisted on seeing her oncologist.

Scans. More imaging. And finally, a CT revealed what laryngitis had been disguising: a tumor wrapped along the lower part of her aorta, pressing against her left vocal cord and paralyzing it. An ENT had missed it. Experience had not.

She needed a thoracic surgeon to biopsy the mass. Sitting there in yet another sterile office, she heard the word *metastatic* float out as just one of several possibilities—maybe it's a benign tumor, maybe it's metastatic breast cancer. The word hung in the air like smoke.

After the biopsy, she gathered friends around her as she waited for the call. This time, she knew you don't get news like that alone if you can help it.

Her oncologist didn't dance around it.

"Carrie, I'm very sorry. We're going to treat you again. It's stage IV metastatic breast cancer."

Same disease. Same HER2 positivity. New home: her aorta. Different category now—no longer "cured" but "incurable," chronic, terminal on paper even if not in spirit.

She was forty.

She had a job she loved.

And this time, she had a two-year-old miracle boy named Nicholas.

Nicholas should not have been medically possible. After years of hormonal suppression and being told her cycle might never return, she'd been stunned to conceive. Twice, she miscarried—once at around four and a half weeks, once at nine. Each loss was its own small funeral.

By the time she saw those two lines a third time, she and her husband Joe didn't tell many people. When she carried Nicholas to term, delivered him via C-section, and held him in her arms in November 2014, she knew exactly what she'd risked by letting hormones flood her system again.

"I don't regret it at all," she says. "He's my blessing."

There are moments, like all mothers with cancer, when she wonders if pregnancy contributed to recurrence. But that question has no clean medical answer, and in her heart, she already knows: she would choose him every time.

The second time around, treatment looked different.

Because the cancer was metastatic, the goal wasn't cure; it was control. Keep the cells quiet. Keep things at bay. Keep her here, and well, for as long as possible.

Aggressive chemo again—but not the same "heavy hitters" as before. Targeted treatments. And then radiation, this time to the mass near the aorta—a therapy her beloved radiologist framed plainly: "There's no solid data I can give you. No percentage. It's basically a 50/50. But it's an option."

This was the same radiologist who had treated her in 2003. The trust was there. Carrie chose to do it. "Let's try to get rid of everything we can," she thought. "If there's a shot, I'm taking it."

Radiation to the chest this time left her throat raw, swallowing nearly impossible, pain severe enough that after eighteen sessions, her team called it. "You've done enough," they said. "You don't need to finish all twenty."

Again, that tension: the part of her that wanted to hit every mark, complete every prescribed session; and the part of her that knew when to say, "Enough. I choose my body over the checklist."

This time, motherhood changed everything.

In 2003, her fear had been almost abstract—*am I going to die? What will my life be?* In 2017, it was acutely concrete: *What happens to Nicholas if I die? Who will read to him? Who will make sure he has a schedule? Who will teach him things the way I would?*

Her husband worked long, physical days as a roofer—out of the house from early morning until dusk in summer. She loved him deeply and knew he loved their son. But she also knew their temperaments were different. "I kind of run the house," she says, not with arrogance but with accuracy. She's the one who manages routines, reading time, playdates, parks, preschool.

"If I'm not here, you can't do it like this," she'd catch herself telling him. Not because he was incapable, but because the idea of Nicholas's life unfolding without her particular brand of structure and nurture was unbearable.

The fear, in those early months, was feral. Every chest pain, every headache, every odd twinge dropped her straight into *this is the end* territory. She'd hold herself together in front of Nicholas, then cry in the shower or in quiet corners where he couldn't see. It wasn't just fear of death; it was fear of leaving chaos behind for her child.

Her village stepped in again, and this time, they stepped in for Nicholas too.

When she needed daily radiation that left her burned and exhausted, her community created a schedule. Two days a week, daycare. The other days? He was scooped up by friends and colleagues and whisked to parks, zoos, playgrounds, swimming pools. Summer adventures, orchestrated by a small army of people who adored him and loved her.

Some days, when she missed him too much and felt well enough, she'd keep him home, prop him up with an iPad and headphones, and let him sit beside her in bed. Not an ideal parenting plan, maybe—but a deeply human one. Sometimes the art of mothering is simply choosing closeness over perfection.

There were days so painful she couldn't speak or swallow, when she stayed with her mom in a small apartment overlooking the water —her mother once again becoming the caregiver who handled the worst of it so Carrie could just be a daughter for a while.

Just when treatment ended and the physical flame began to cool, her friends at Children's Hospital and beyond did something extraordinary: they organized a banquet.

In May 2017, still bald, bloated from steroids, and raw from radiation, she walked into a hall filled with more than four hundred people—college friends, gym families, coworkers, relatives, and strangers who only knew that "Carrie needs us." There were raffles, donations, speeches. They raised enough money for her to take a full year off work to heal and stay home with Nicholas.

It was humbling, overwhelming, and deeply clarifying. Community wasn't just a nice idea; it was survival. Their generosity gave her time—time to let her body recover, time to establish a new normal, time to be present with her son.

The year that followed was not some serene convalescence. It was messy and hard. She was exhausted, often running herself ragged on the good days because she was so grateful to be able to do *anything* at all. She wrestled with PTSD, flashbacks, and that old terror every time her body made a noise she didn't understand. And as friends she'd met in online metastatic groups began to die, survivor's guilt crept in.

"They have little kids too," she'd think. "Why am I still here and they're not?"

Blessed. That was the word that kept surfacing. Not in a hashtag way, but in a stunned, reverent way.

Somewhere in all this, acceptance began to take shape—not as surrender, but as a kind of grounded clarity.

She learned the rhythm of metastatic life: scans every three months; treatments every three weeks or thirty days. She learned that her infusion chair could be, strangely, a place of rest—a warm blanket, a needle in her port, and ninety minutes where no one could ask her for anything. A forced pause in which she could answer emails, listen to music, or simply sleep.

She found, for a while, a metastatic support group fifteen to thirty minutes from home—a circle of women who truly understood the terrain she was walking. When that group dissolved, it left a jagged hole. Online groups helped—HER2-positive groups, metastatic community forums—but they came with their own heartbreak as profile photos turned to memorial posts.

At home, Joe coped in the way many partners do: by not talking much about the thing that scared him most. "He's there for me," she says. "He helps. But we don't really sit and process it together." Friends point out that he's probably more afraid than he lets on. It's something they may still need support for, in time.

With Nicholas, she walks a careful, intentional line.

He has always known her as a mother with scars, a port in her chest, and frequent doctor visits. When he was smaller and their bodies still shared space in the bathroom and shower, he'd touch the scar on her breast or the bump of her port and say, "That's where you get your medicine."

The question of what to say and how much to tell him haunted her. Advice from pediatricians and social workers trickled in slowly; there was no ready-made, local program for "Mom has metastatic cancer and a preschooler." Finally, Dana-Farber sent a packet—a children's coloring book designed to help explain parental illness in age-appropriate doses.

One day, she sat down with Nicholas and opened to page one: a simple picture of a parent driving a car with a child in the backseat.

"We go to the doctor's a lot, don't we?" she said.

"Yeah," he nodded.

She explained, gently, that she had something called cancer, and the doctors were giving her medicine to help her body work better.

Just that. One page. One small truth.

Afterward, she felt like thirty pounds had been lifted off her shoulders. She didn't need to dump the whole story on him; she just needed to be honest at his level, and let questions come when they came.

Now, at five, he knows: "Mommy has cancer. She goes to the doctor for medicine." As he grows, the pages of that coloring book will turn, and the story will deepen.

There are still hard, heavy days. Days when exhaustion sends her back to bed after school drop-off, and she battles the voice that says she should be doing laundry instead of sleeping. Days when survivor's guilt flares. Days when Nicholas says or does something so gloriously ordinary that her heart aches with the awareness of how fragile this all is.

But there's also this:

She has learned to love routine—not as a prison, but as a scaffolding.

She has learned to accept help without apology.

She has learned that sometimes being a good mother means letting your kid watch cartoons while you lie next to them, because being near is the most you can offer and also the thing that matters most.

And she has learned that strength isn't just what you show the world. It's also the way you allow yourself to fall apart in the shower, then dry your face, step out, and pack a preschool lunch.

Carrie may have stepped away from the hospital floor and the chaos of trauma codes, but the heart she used there—the one that can witness unimaginable pain and still show up with compassion—hasn't gone anywhere. She's channeling it now into her home, her friendships, and the way she shows up for others with metastatic disease.

This is the life she is creating in the in-between: not before cancer, not after cancer, but *with* cancer. A life stitched together with little boy giggles, preschool schedules, infusion appointments, and a village that refuses to let her carry this alone.

It is not the life she would have chosen.

But it is, undeniably, a life—hers—and she is still here, holding on and letting go, one day at a time.

Closing Reflection

There's a particular courage that belongs to people living with metastatic disease. It's not the cinematic, triumphant kind. It's quieter, more complicated: the courage to build a life you love in a body that keeps reminding you of its limits.

Carrie's story shows us that art is not only something you hang on a wall. It's how you shape a day. It's how you braid gratitude into ordinary hours—school pick-ups, library trips, infusion appointments, bedtime snuggles. It's how you hold your child's future in one hand and your own fear in the other and decide, again and again, to keep loving, keep showing up, keep planning for tomorrow.

Canvas of Courage

The art of holding on and letting go is not about choosing one or the other. It's about learning to do both at once: holding on to hope, community, and the fierce joy of being Nicholas's mom, while letting go of old timelines, old definitions of "healthy," and the fantasy that certainty is something we're ever guaranteed.

She taught us that courage does not roar.
Sometimes it whispers through routine,
through showing up on days when energy is thin
and love must do the heavy lifting.
Since our interview in 2020, Carrie has passed away.
She died peacefully, surrounded by those who loved her.
And still —
this is not where her story ends.
Because what remains is not her diagnosis.
What remains is her devotion.
Her tenderness.
Her discipline of choosing life inside uncertainty.
What remains is a mother who showed her son
how to live fully, even while dying.
What remains is proof that embracing cancer
does not mean accepting defeat —
it means refusing to abandon yourself
while walking through the unimaginable.
Carrie continues
in the routines she modeled,
in the love she poured into her child,
in the women who will read her story
and feel less alone.
Her body may have rested,
but her impact did not.
And that, too, is an art.

. . .

Carrie's Grace Notes

- **Let people be your village.**
    - You don't have to do it all. You *cannot* do it all. Let the friend take your toddler to the zoo. Let the neighbor cook. Let the banquet happen. The art is in receiving as much as in giving.
- **Routines are medicine, too.**
    - School drop-off times, nap windows, radiation appointments, bedtime stories—these become anchors. In a body and life that feel unpredictable, rhythm is a kind of therapy.
- **You're allowed to have a breakdown—as long as you remember to stand back up.**
    - Carrie cries in the shower, in her mom's apartment, in quiet places where she can let fear roar. Then she wipes her face and keeps going. You don't have to be stoic to be strong.
- **"Good enough" counts.**
    - Some days, the perfect playdate gets replaced by an iPad and headphones. Some dinners are cereal. Some "activities" are just lying in bed together. Presence matters more than Pinterest.
- **Use age-appropriate honesty with your kids.**
    - Small truths, one page at a time. "Mommy has cancer." "These doctors give me medicine." You don't have to unload the whole story at once. You just have to be trustworthy.
- **Find people who *get it*.**
    - Online groups, metastatic circles, even one other parent walking a similar path—these connections matter. They normalize your fears, offer practical tips, and remind you you're not alone.

- **Scanxiety and survivor's guilt are real.**
  - Expect them. Name them. It doesn't mean you're ungrateful; it means you're human. Talk about it—with a therapist, a trusted friend, or others in the metastatic community.
- **Reframe the infusion chair.**
  - Instead of seeing treatment days only as punishment, notice what they also give you: enforced rest, a warm blanket, 90 minutes where the only thing on your to-do list is to receive.
- **Let work and identity evolve.**
  - Leaving a job you love can feel like another loss—but it can also open space for a different kind of vocation. Right now, Carrie's full-time job is mothering and healing. That is enough.
- **You are not a failure for needing rest.**
  - If your body sends you back to bed after drop-off, listen. Rest is not laziness; it is repair. Your worth is not measured in tasks checked off.

The Art of Becoming Unbreakable
Melanie's Story

W＊*hen life split her open, she learned to remake herself in colors stronger than fear.*

Every portrait begins with contrast. Light against dark. Color blooming through shadow. In the creative act—just as in healing—we paint with what remains after the breaking. Melanie's story reminds me that even the deepest fractures can become fault lines for beauty.

Melanie's journey is not one of quiet endurance — it is a story of collision, shattering, and fierce reconstruction. Hers is the art of breaking open and rebuilding, the art of resilience forged in the body, in motherhood, and in the raw edges of uncertainty. What she survived did not soften her. It sculpted her. And it taught her that sometimes the masterpiece is not who we were before, but who we become because we were tested.

When we first spoke, I could sense in her voice the strength of someone who has stared into uncertainty and chosen grace anyway. She lives her life like a mixed-media canvas—layer upon layer of faith, humor, heartbreak, and courage. Through her, I was reminded that art and gratitude share the same purpose: to turn pain into presence, and to keep creating even when the picture changes.

Living Courageously with Cancer

Melanie was only thirty-four when the word "leukemia" entered her vocabulary and changed her life's palette overnight. A hallway phone call from her oncologist—*you have chronic myeloid leukemia*—shattered her ordinary evening at work. Her grandfather had died from leukemia years earlier; to her, the word meant death. She was a new mother, her son barely a year old, and the news felt like being dropped into darkness without a map.

Yet somewhere in that darkness, she began sketching a new kind of strength.

Medication placed the disease into remission, and she learned to coexist with fear. But just when color returned to her world, life added another bold stroke: stage III breast cancer in 2011. A mastectomy, 14 lymph nodes removed, chemotherapy, radiation, Tamoxifen. The rhythm of treatment replaced the rhythm of ordinary life. "I just kept going," she told me. "Because stopping wasn't an option."

For several years, she tried to live in remission's fragile light. Then, in 2018, the cancer returned—this time stage IV, metastasized to her hip and arm. She began estrogen blockers, injections, and a regimen of medication she half-jokingly called her "chemical cocktail." There were side effects, fatigue, pain, and flashes of menopause before her time. But there was also laughter, resilience, and a rebellious refusal to let disease define her.

"I just do it," she said simply. "I have to. I have a son, three dogs, a family that needs me. You don't realize how strong you are until you don't have a choice."

The Weight and the Wings

During her first diagnosis, Melanie was far from family. Her husband battled his own medical issues; her work environment questioned her illness; the isolation was crushing. But when she was re-diagnosed, she moved back home to Baltimore, closer to her parents and sister. This time, support came flooding in. She moved in with her parents during chemotherapy so she could focus on survival while they cared for her young son. Her sister became weekend childcare; her husband packed up their Ohio home. A network of love became her scaffolding.

"I couldn't have done it without them," she said. "They drugged me just so I could sleep through the worst of it. And they never let me feel alone."

Today, Melanie still works full-time, balancing her stage IV diagnosis with caring for her now 14-year-old son with autism. Her life is a study in motion—grace under constant revision. Some days are painted in pain; others shimmer with humor and defiance. She jokes about "chemo brain" and losing her cat bowl, about crying over a missing couch receipt and then laughing through the meltdown. Her laughter is medicine. Her dark humor, a brushstroke of rebellion against despair.

"If you don't laugh at it, the horror of it will eat you alive," she told me. "Sometimes you have to make fun of yourself just to stay human."

Finding the Gift Inside the Grief

When asked if cancer had given her anything positive, Melanie paused. Then she said something that has echoed in me ever since:
"I don't put things on hold anymore."

Since her stage IV diagnosis, Melanie has given herself permission to live loudly. She buys the perfume, the makeup, the cat. She drives four hours for dinner because she wants the experience, not the excuse. She takes road trips with her sister, adopts stray joy like a rescue animal. She laughs about collecting "three dogs and a cat too many," but beneath the humor is a deeper truth: every living thing in her home is a heartbeat she refuses to take for granted.

Her aunt and father both passed within months of each other, amplifying her awareness of time's fragility. "After that," she said, "I just stopped waiting. I wanted to live while I still could."

To Melanie, gratitude isn't passive. It's a daily art form—an act of rebellion against the statistics. She has learned to paint joy over fear, to collage humor onto hardship, to sculpt courage from exhaustion. Her masterpiece isn't the absence of struggle; it's the decision to keep creating through it.

The Courage to Share

Melanie believes sharing stories is a responsibility. "By telling my story, maybe someone else feels less alone," she said. When she first joined online support groups, she found answers that even her doctors missed—side effects dismissed as 'impossible,' symptoms others quietly endured. She found relief in community, truth in shared experience. Now she pays that forward daily, guiding newly diagnosed patients toward resources, research, and courage.

Her advocacy is quiet but constant. She believes in honesty—telling people you're sick, letting them see the reality, because silence only breeds shame. "Don't pretend everything's fine when it isn't," she said. "Ask for help. Tell your job. Tell your friends. You can't do this alone."

That raw transparency is part of her art. It takes courage to be seen in the unfinished stages of healing—to say *here I am, work in progress and still beautiful.*

Closing Reflection

Melanie's story is a portrait of resilience painted in unfiltered color. Her life—like art—is not about perfection but process. Each diagnosis, each scar, each moment of laughter in a doctor's office adds another layer to her canvas. Through her, I am reminded that the act of living is itself an art form—a daily choice to keep painting when the surface cracks.

In gratitude, we find texture. In vulnerability, we find light. And in stories like Melanie's, we see that the strongest artworks are not those that hide their wounds but those that transform them into something unbreakable.

Melanie's Grace Notes

- **Be your own advocate.** Ask questions. If something feels off, trust your instincts and seek second opinions.
- **Find your support system.** Family, friends, online groups—community is lifesaving.
- **Be honest about your diagnosis.** Transparency builds understanding and reduces isolation.
- **Prioritize energy, not appearance.** Choose self-care over housework and perfection.

- **Laugh at the absurdity.** Dark humor and self-deprecation are powerful coping tools.
- **Create your new normal.** Accept change and find joy within it—life does not pause for fear.
- **Share your story.** Your voice may save someone else's life or light their path through darkness.
- **Embrace the now.** Buy the cat, take the trip, eat the dessert. Gratitude is art in motion.

The Healing Science of Art

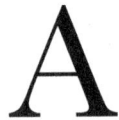 gentle fusion of artistic expression and somatic regulation.

Long before science learned how to measure it, humans understood this truth intuitively:
art heals.
We carved symbols into cave walls.
We sang while working.
We danced to grieve, to celebrate, to survive.
Creativity has always been medicine — not as decoration, but as regulation, connection, and meaning-making.
Only recently has science caught up to what the body has always known.

What Happens in the Body When We Create

. . .

When a person is facing illness, especially cancer, the body often lives in a state of prolonged stress. The nervous system remains on high alert — scanning, bracing, preparing. This survival mode is useful in short bursts, but harmful when sustained over time.

Research now shows that engaging in creative practices can interrupt this cycle.

When we create — whether through drawing, painting, writing, music, or movement — the brain shifts out of fight-or-flight and into a parasympathetic state. This is the state associated with rest, digestion, healing, and repair.

Studies have shown that:

- Viewing or creating art can lower cortisol (the body's primary stress hormone)
- Heart rate and blood pressure decrease during creative engagement
- The immune system responds more favorably when stress is reduced
- Emotional processing becomes more accessible and less overwhelming

In simple terms:
art tells the nervous system it is safe to exhale.

And for someone living inside a medical diagnosis, that exhale matters.

Art as Regulation, Not Distraction

There is a common misconception that art is a way to "escape" reality. In healing spaces, the opposite is true.

Art does not remove pain — it creates a container for it.

Creative practices allow emotions to move through the body rather than lodge inside it. Fear, grief, anger, and uncertainty find expression without requiring explanation. For people who are exhausted from talking about their illness, art offers a language beyond words.

This is not avoidance.

This is integration.

Neuroscience shows that when sensory input (color, texture, movement, rhythm) is introduced, the brain engages in bilateral processing — allowing emotional material to be held without overwhelming the system. This is why many people report feeling calmer, clearer, or unexpectedly lighter after creative sessions, even when difficult emotions surface.

Healing does not always arrive as relief.

Sometimes it arrives as release.

The Difference Between Art Therapy and Therapeutic Art

It is important to clarify a distinction that often gets blurred.

Art Therapy is a licensed clinical practice used to treat mental health diagnoses. It is guided by trained clinicians and operates within therapeutic frameworks.

Therapeutic art and arts-in-health practices, however, are not about diagnosis or treatment. They are about well-being.

These practices create space for:

- Emotional expression without interpretation
- Regulation of the nervous system
- Reconnection to self beyond illness
- Restoration of agency and choice
- Meaning-making during uncertainty

You do not need to be "good" at art.
You do not need to understand what you make.
You only need to show up.
The healing happens in the doing.

Why This Matters During Illness

Cancer is not only a physical experience. It is psychological, emotional, relational, and spiritual. Treatment protocols are designed to address the body — but often leave the inner world unattended.

Creative practices help fill that gap.

They return choice to people who have lost control over their schedules, their bodies, and sometimes their identities. They allow patients, survivors, and caregivers to reconnect with something untouched by diagnosis.

In a hospital setting, art can:

- Restore a sense of humanity
- Reduce feelings of isolation
- Create moments of presence inside uncertainty
- Help patients process experiences that are too heavy for language

Art does not promise cure.
It offers care.

What the Research Tells Us

. . .

Multiple studies across oncology, psychology, and neuroscience support the integration of creative practices into healthcare environments.

Research published by the World Health Organization and leading medical institutions has found that arts-based interventions can:

- Reduce anxiety and depression
- Improve patient experience and satisfaction
- Support emotional resilience
- Enhance quality of life during and after treatment

But beyond the data lies something just as important:
People feel seen again.
And feeling seen changes everything.

Healing Is Not the Absence of Pain

Art does not make illness fair.
It does not erase loss.
It does not offer easy answers.
What it does offer is companionship.
A reminder that even in uncertainty, creation is still possible. Expression is still allowed. Beauty can still exist alongside fear.
Healing, in this context, is not about returning to who you were before.
It is about learning how to live — honestly, gently, courageously — inside what is.
And sometimes, the most powerful medicine is not something administered,

but something remembered:
That you are still human.
Still creative.
Still whole.

An Invitation to Create

You don't need to be an artist to be here.

You don't need talent, training, or the right words. You only need breath, presence, and permission. If you're holding this book, something inside you is already listening. Creation is not about producing something beautiful. It is about allowing something true to surface.

So before you turn the page—before you rush toward meaning or closure—pause.

Place one hand on your body. Anywhere that feels safe. Your chest. Your stomach. Your thigh. Feel that you are here.

. . .

Canvas of Courage

This book is not asking you to fix yourself. It is asking you to notice yourself. The stories you've read are layered with courage, grief, resilience, tenderness, and grace. They may have stirred memories you didn't expect. They may have opened doors you thought were closed. They may have softened you—or shaken you. That is not a mistake. That is the work.

Creation is one of the oldest ways humans metabolize experience. Before language was refined, we marked walls. Before therapy existed, we sang, danced, carved, stitched, and traced meaning with our hands. You are allowed to do the same.

This invitation is simple:

- To draw without knowing what will appear.
- To write without worrying if it makes sense.
- To move your body in response to emotion.
- To sit quietly and let an image form.
- To choose color based on feeling, not logic.

There is no right way to respond to what you're carrying.
There is only *your* way.
You may feel resistance.
You may feel nothing at all.
You may feel too much.
All of it belongs.
If you choose to create, do it gently.
Light a candle.
Play music that feels safe.
Set a timer if that helps contain the experience.
Stop whenever you need to.
And if today is not the day to create—
that is also part of healing.

Nerissa Balland

Sometimes the most powerful act is simply witnessing what has already been made visible inside you.

Let this book be a companion, not a demand.
Let these stories walk beside you, not ahead of you.
Let your own voice arrive when it is ready.
Creation is not about becoming someone new.
It is about remembering who you already are.
And if nothing else, let this be true:
You are allowed to take up space.
You are allowed to feel deeply.
You are allowed to create meaning from what you've survived.
This is not the end of the story.
It is an opening.
Take your time.

What We Carry Forward

We do not leave these stories behind.

They stay with us—
    in the body,
    in the breath,
    in the quiet moments without asking.

Each woman carried something different:
    a diagnosis spoken too quickly,
    children held close while fear waited nearby,
    a body altered, a future rewritten.
    And yet what lingers is not only what was lost.
    It is what remained.
    A courage that did not need to be loud.
    A strength that looked like showing up again.
    A love so steady it learned how to live inside uncertainty.

Healing, we learn, is not a finish line.
    It is a relationship.

What We Carry Forward

One that changes shape as we do.
Some women healed in visible ways.
Some healed quietly, in places no one could see.
Some are no longer here—
and still, their lives speak.
They speak through the children they loved.
Through the choices they made.
Through the uncertainty.

If you recognized yourself anywhere in these pages,
    let this be your permission to pause.
    You do not need to be brave today.
    You do not need to be grateful.
    You do not need to understand yet.
    It is enough to be here.
    It is enough to breathe.
    It is enough to carry this gently.

Healing is not something you earn.
    It arrives when you stop abandoning yourself.
    When you allow rest to be part of survival.
    When you let tenderness coexist with strength.
    May you trust the wisdom of your body.
    May you honor the pace of your heart.
    May you know—deeply and without question—
    that nothing about you is broken.
    You are becoming.
    And you are held as you do.
    To live awake.
    To love deeply.
    To create meaning where you can.
    And to remember the women who showed us how.

What We Carry Forward

We carry them forward
    in the way we choose presence over perfection,
    connection over fear,
    and honesty over silence.
    Their stories do not end here.
    Neither does yours.
    Close the book when you're ready.
    But don't rush.
    Some things are meant to stay with you.

About the Author

Nerissa Balland is an artist, mother, and two-time cancer survivor whose life and work live at the intersection of creativity, healing, and truth.

Her journey into the world of therapeutic art did not begin in a classroom or a certification program — it began in survival. In 2016, while five months pregnant, Nerissa was diagnosed with metastatic melanoma. What followed was a season of impossible choices, profound fear, and radical awakening. Cancer dismantled the life she had carefully built and revealed the one she had quietly abandoned.

Trained as a visual artist with a Master of Fine Arts in Painting from Pratt Institute, Nerissa spent nearly two decades working in marketing, branding, and design before cancer forced her to confront a question many women postpone until it is unavoidable: *What am I doing with the time I have?*

Art became her lifeline long before it became her mission.

Through layered texture, symbolism, movement, and color, she began to heal parts of herself that language could not reach. What started as personal expression evolved into purpose — and eventually into service. Today, Nerissa is an Arts-in-Health and Therapeutic Arts Practitioner who combines visual art, neuroscience, mindfulness, coaching, and creative facilitation to support individuals navigating illness, trauma, and profound life transitions.

Her work is grounded in both lived experience and science. She holds advanced training in Therapeutic Arts, Neurolinguistic Programming, Cognitive Behavioral Therapy, and Rational Emotive

Behavioral Therapy, and has facilitated creative wellness workshops for hospitals, cancer centers, universities, schools, and community organizations. Yet it is not credentials that shape her work — it is listening.

As a mother of two young sons conceived through IVF, Nerissa understands the layered complexity of caregiving while healing, of holding fear and love in the same breath, of showing up when the body feels uncertain. Her work is informed by this reality: that healing is not linear, strength is not performative, and joy is not a luxury — it is a responsibility.

This book was born from a simple but radical act: making space for women to tell the truth about their lives without being rushed, reframed, or fixed. These stories are not meant to inspire through perfection. They are meant to witness, to validate, and to remind the reader that even in the presence of illness, life remains textured, meaningful, and profoundly human.

Nerissa lives and works in South Florida, where she continues to create, exhibit, and sell her art. She lead workshops, and build spaces where healing is allowed to look different for everyone.

She believes that sometimes the greatest challenge we face awakens the opportunity to become our greatest gift — and that art, in all its forms, can help us remember who we are when everything else falls away.

Acknowledgments

This book exists because women said yes—
  yes to remembering,
  yes to revisiting moments they had long tucked away,
  yes to telling the truth even when it trembled in their throats.
  To the mothers who shared their stories in these pages:
  thank you for trusting me.
  Thank you for your honesty, your vulnerability, your humor, your rage, your faith, your exhaustion, your hope.
  You did not offer polished narratives—
  you offered your hearts.
  This book belongs to you.
  To the women whose stories do not continue beyond these pages,
  but whose presence is still deeply felt:
  you are not forgotten.
  Your love, your courage, and your way of moving through this world live on—
  in your children, in the people you changed, and in every reader who carries you forward now.
  To the families, partners, children, and caregivers—
  the quiet warriors behind the scenes—
  thank you for holding space, holding hands, holding homes together when everything felt uncertain.
  Your love made survival possible.
  Your steadiness mattered more than you know.
  To my own family—

my husband, Michael, for standing beside me with patience, humor, and unwavering belief,
and my children, Eli & Teddy, who unknowingly taught me how to live more awake, more honestly, more presently—
you are my reason, my grounding, my joy.
Everything I create is touched by you.

To the healers, guides, doctors, therapists, coaches, spiritual leaders, and artists who walked alongside me and these women—thank you for reminding us that healing is not only physical, that listening is a form of medicine, and that humanity must never be lost in the process of care.

Thank you to my medical team, who without fail have been my saving grace: Dr. Lawrence A. Schiffman, Dr. Brian J. Katz, Dr. Jose Lutzky, Dr. Juan C. Paramo, and Jeanelle S. King, PA-C.

To the creative practices that held us when words failed—art, movement, breath, prayer, silence—thank you for making space where fear softened and truth could emerge.

And finally, to you—the reader—
if you found your way here, know this:
you are not alone.
Whether you are grieving, surviving, supporting, or simply learning how to hold life more gently,
your presence completes this book.
Thank you for listening.
Thank you for witnessing.
Thank you for carrying these stories forward.

www.ingramcontent.com/pod-product-compliance
Lightning Source LLC
Chambersburg PA
CBHW020540030426
42337CB00013B/924